WI MASKS WILL KILL YOU

A journey into science and ethics

Lucia
Bruno

First published in Great Britain in 2022 by atmayantra publishing

Copyright © 2022 by Lucia Isabella Carla Bruno
Cover Image by Mathew Schwart
Formatting by The Amethyst Angel

ISBN: 978-1-7391569-4-7

The moral right of the authors has been asserted.

First Edition

ACKNOWLEDGEMENTS

I wish to thank my partner Michael John Christian and my daughters Luna and Alice Motola for the constant help, support, and encouragement. Specifically, Michael for editing, graphic design input and insights, Luna for offering to translate the book into Spanish, Alice for editing, providing scientific considerations and offering a translation into Italian. Pilar Cecilia Montes Bori for friendship and hard work in designing most of the pictures, the initial formatting and graphic design. Michelle Gordon for the final graphic design and formatting and assisting me in self-publishing the book.

I am honoured for Stephen Petty to have written a foreword and for his comments on the chapter dedicated to his work: a relentless and constant effort to prove that masks do not work. My gratitude goes also to each and every author and scientist who wrote and researched this subject and gave me the knowledge to even conceive the idea to write this book. You are all mentioned in my reference list and I tried to quote you as much as I was able to.

Thank you to my cat Blackie for sitting on my manuscript in approval.

I also would like to acknowledge NHS100K, TOGETHER, Smile Free and Workers of England Union for their campaigns to bring evidence-based science back to the centre of many critical issues.

CONTENTS

FOREWORD

This book titled, *Wearing Masks Will Kill You* by Lucia Isabella Carla Bruno, is an excellent introduction to the harms done by masks and face coverings as they are more formally referred to. With tens-of-millions of dollars spent by Governmental and NGO organisations using the powerful psychological tools of persuasion i) fear, ii) emotional appeal, and iii) propaganda of repeated message to convince company leaders, local and regional authorities, and the public of the benefits of wearing masks or face coverings, it is little wonder the public is so compliant and confused.

The hill to overcome this real misinformation is great, but a handful of scientists, including those in the relevant field of industrial hygiene, have spoken out regarding the nonsense and harms of masking and many in the public are beginning to understand they have been misled. This book provides you with information that supports many of you whose natural intuition is that masks or face coverings cannot and do not protect one from infectious diseases and introduces you to real engineering solutions [dilution (more fresh air), filtration, and destruction] that have been available since 1950, that actually work and have been largely ignored during this pandemic.

Stephen Petty, P.E., C.I.H., C.S.P.

INTRODUCTION

"Those who can make you believe absurdities can make you commit atrocities." – Francois Marie Arouet de Voltaire

"The importance of breathing need hardly be stressed. It provides the oxygen for the metabolic processes; literally it supports the fires of life. But breath as "pneuma" is also the spirit or soul. We live in an ocean of air like fish in a body of water. By our breathing we are attuned to our atmosphere. If we inhibit our breathing we isolate ourselves from the medium in which we exist. In all Oriental and mystic philosophies, the breath holds the secret to the highest bliss.
That is why breathing is the dominant factor in the practice of Yoga."
– Alexander Lowen, The Voice of the Body

This book is born out of a wound. On the 24th of July 2020 the UK government mandated mask wearing in any public venue. This became an even stricter rule in the NHS. The acute mental health ward in which I was employed at that time adopted and enforced the same legislation. Being a qualified yoga teacher since 1994, this was not sitting well with me at all. I had plenty of theoretical and practical reasons to deem this as a very unhealthy and unscientific measure. Nevertheless, I reluctantly complied, as did many other employees: I have a mortgage to pay and my highest dream is for me and my family not to die of starvation. In July 2021, after exactly a year of constant mask wearing, up to fourteen hours, virtually every day, I contracted what in layman terms is called 'Mask Mouth': bleeding and receding gums, excruciating and recurring painful ulcers, extensive pus production, wobbly teeth moving out of place in any possible direction, malodorous breath.

I was ridiculed for suggesting that the cause of my issue was surgical mask wearing. I was then targeted, bullied, accused of unprofessional conduct and various other allegations if I was seen removing my mask even only for few seconds. Exemption was not a consented option if I was to remain in a patient facing role. This, despite the fact that patients, whether positive for COVID or otherwise had no requirement to wear a mask or a face covering. Apparently ill patients do not spread infections, healthy staff do.

In September 2021, I went to see a specialist doctor with so many qualifications after her name I could fill an A4 page. She just confirmed my own diagnosis: management induced stress and surgical mask wearing were the culprits of my problem.

When I reported the doctor's medical opinion, management thought I had gone to some quack consultant in 'Hippy land' and they required me to go through an official Occupational Health assessment. I met this requirement in December 2021 and low and behold, the Occupational Health nurse just repeated verbatim the same words used by the specialist doctor.

She wrote a detailed report and during our meeting she said:

'Masks are designed for surgical settings, not for any other use. In surgical settings they are normally used for no more than few hours continuously. Nobody should be asked to use a surgical mask for prolonged amounts of time and without providing regular and planned breaks. Surgical masks should be used only when necessary and when in direct contact with patients. Masks have a repellent and impermeable coating that traps CO_2 and bacteria and cause several health problems. By now everybody should know this very well and especially management and the infection control lead.'

My line manager ignored the above all together and said I could not continue working in the ward if I could not wear a surgical mask at all times. I later on discovered, too late I must add, that this was plainly unlawful under UK employment legislation and certainly discriminatory. Nevertheless, I was redeployed and ping-ponged between various other wards and hospitals. More targeting, bullying, accusation of unprofessional conduct and various other allegations were following me at any new location.

At this point I had two main choices: remain a silent victim of the system or become a wounded healer and help other people in similar circumstances.

The concept of wounded healer has its roots in mythology and in ancient shamanic practices. In recent times, psychologist Carl Jung reinstated this archetypal figure in his body of work. In a nutshell, a wounded healer is someone that has gone through a trauma or an illness and is better equipped to understand and heal others through "heightened patience, empathy and acceptance". Wounded healers do not pontificate out of hearsay, they have gone through the ordeal themselves and somehow managed to have a breakthrough rather than a breakdown.

In Greek mythology, the centaur Chiron was the first known archetype of a wounded Healer. Heracles had accidentally hit him with an arrow dipped in the poisonous blood of Hydra. Chiron was immortal and could not die but was suffering excruciating pain. Chiron, from that day on, kept healing the sick and the injured.

My illness and the various abuses that I had to endure, drove me into research and gave me the motivation to explore this subject in depth, starting from the mere physical, moving to the emotional, psychological, social, sociological and spiritual spheres.

In the past two years I have been studying at University level and for that reason I have had access to the best evidence based and peer reviewed literature.

This book is my personal journey into scientific findings and ethical reflections.

The title of this work is at the same time strong and factual. The aim is to finally provide some evidence based science to counteract the misinformation that many had to endure on a daily basis when self-appointed experts, after armchair crash courses in virology, were falsely affirming that if someone would not wear a surgical mask their patients, themselves and grandma were going to get COVID and die. The opposite, as a matter of fact, is actually true. Mask wearers produce and spread far more infected COVID particles than maskless individuals. Fact. They rebreathe this amplified viral load deeper in their lungs and have at least 50% more chances to get infected and die.

This work is here to prove this, among many other facts and it is also my little contribution to other people that had to go through similar tribulations and are still confused and wounded.

Let's dive in.

CHAPTER ONE

Brief history of breathing

"Then the Lord God formed the man from the dust of the ground and breathed into his nostrils the breath of life, and the man became a living being." – Genesis 2:7

In the beginning of the Earth's history, our atmosphere contained very little oxygen. The first rise of this element came about in the GOE, the Great Oxygenation Event at the start of the Proterozoic era, about 2,500 million years ago. The increase to modern levels of oxygen (around 21%) happened during the Phanerozoic era that started 540 million years ago.

Respiration begun in the oceans around 400 million years ago.

Fish developed gills as a means of more efficiently absorbing the oxygen contained in water. This gave these primordial ancestors a significant increase in energy levels and the ability to grow and evolve more rapidly.

The next step was for amphibians to gradually move out of the sea and start breathing air. Gills progressively transformed into lungs. Birds, reptiles and mammals further perfected breathing in the next evolutionary phase.

Every improvement in breathing was followed by a step up in evolution and a better chance of survival. Eventually, human beings became one of the products of this elaborate process. Further on in history, ancient civilisations started to reflect and examine the functions and meaning of respiration. For a very long time, the spiritual essence of breathing was the primary aspect of this human experience with the physical being a secondary and trivial component.

Breath and breathing also had a very important role in philosophy, mythology, cosmology, rituals and spiritual practice. Various breathing techniques were used for religious and healing purposes as links between nature, the human body, the psyche, and the spirit.

For millennia shamans, priests and yogi used breathing to expand their consciousness, control their emotions and minds and ultimately progress on their spiritual path. They strongly believed that illness is mostly caused by incorrect and shallow breathing.

For example, in Sanskrit and Pali the word सुख (sukha) represents happiness, pleasure, ease, joy or bliss. Etymologically it is composed of 'su', which means happy and positive and 'kha': breath. All together sukha means 'who that breathes correctly'. दुख (duhkha), on the contrary, means suffering, unhappiness, pain, unsatisfactory and stress. Etymologically it is composed of 'duh' or bad and negative and 'kha': breath representing 'who that breathes incorrectly'.

The very same happens in the native Hawaiian tradition and medicine in which the word 'ha' means the divine spirit, wind, air, and breath. It is contained in the popular Hawaiian 'aloha' expression that is used in many different contexts. It is usually translated as presence 'alo' of the Divine Breath 'ha'. Its opposite, 'ha'ole', meaning literally 'without breath' or 'without life', is a term that native Hawaiians have applied to describe the white-skinned foreigners that arrived with James Cook in 1778 and thereafter.

It comes as no surprise that breathing supports physical, emotional, mental and spiritual wellbeing and consequently life itself.

In ancient Greece it was believed that through breathing living beings would inhale 'pneuma' or "aithein" (ether), the spiritual essences of life.

The Greeks also saw breath as being closely related to the psyche. The word 'phren' was used both for diaphragm and mind (for example in the term schizophrenia which literally means split mind).

In many languages, the word for breath and spirit are the same. In Greek, the word 'pneuma', in Latin 'spiritus', in traditional Chinese medicine, the word 'chi', in Japan 'ki', in Hebrew 'ruac', in Arabic 'rouh' that also means wind, inspiration, rest, relaxation, going home and happiness. In Slavic languages, spirit and breath have the same linguistic root too.

In Sanskrit, 'prana' means breath, life force and vital energy. In yoga, pranayama is the expansion of the life force, and practitioners, through direct experience, know that expanding breathing expands life energy.

Qigong, that originated in China around 2,000 B.C., means cultivation of life energy through movement, breathing exercises and meditation. In this context too, correct respiration provides vitality and healing.

The same conclusions were reached in other religious and spiritual disciplines such as Taoism, Buddhism, Hinduism, early Christianity, Shamanism, Sufism, and many martial arts.

Specific techniques involving intense breathing or withholding of breath are also part of various exercises in Kundalini Yoga, Siddha Yoga, the Tibetan Vajrayana, Sufi practice, Burmese Buddhist and Taoist meditation, the Balinese monkey chant or Ketjak, the Inuit Eskimo throat music, Tibetan and Mongolian multi-vocal chanting, and singing of kirtans, bhajans and Sufi chants.

In Buddhism, Anāpānasati is a basic form of meditation that literally means "mindfulness of breathing". According to the Anāpānasati Sutra, practicing this form of meditation leads to nirvana, a transcendent state in which there is no pain, desire, or identity and the individual is liberated from the effects of karma and the cycle of death and rebirth. Nirvana is the ultimate aim of Buddhism.

Cultivation of special attention to breathing represents also an essential part of certain Taoist and Christian practices. For example, the original form of baptism practiced by the Essenes involved forced submersion of the initiate under water for an extended period of time. This resulted in a powerful experience of death and rebirth. Following the same concept, in some other groups, the neophytes were choked by smoke, strangulation, or compression of the carotid arteries.

In the West the approach to breathing started under a similar conceptual basis but later on took a completely different direction: breathing lost its sacred meaning and was deprived of its connection to psyche and spirit.

In mediaeval times we see the first treatments of respiratory disorders with herbs and potions under the promise that illness of the lungs had an organic basis and was caused by imbalance in the homeostasis of the body.

During the Renaissance Leonardo da Vinci explored the anatomy of the human body in great detail. This new approach promoted the advancement of medicine and at the same time, started the separation of the spiritual and physical aspect of respiration.

Western medicine reduced it to a mere important physiological function. With the invention of the microscope in the late sixteenth century, Marcello Malpighi observed and described the structure of the lungs of several frogs. Other scientist studied other phenomena such as air pressure in relation to volume, or examined the physics and chemistry of our atmosphere with the realisation that it consisted of a mixture of different gases. After the industrial revolution human beings had to face air pollution and its consequences on the respiratory system.

In the last few decades, however, Western therapists have rediscovered the healing potential of breath and have developed techniques that utilise it.

Despite scepticism, in the twentieth century, different breathing methods, mostly derived from yoga, have been developed, explored and applied under the name of 'breathwork'. Christina and Stanislav Grof (one of the founders of Transpersonal Psychology) developed Holotropic Breathwork, a method of psychotherapy that uses fast breathing, music and specific exercises to explore altered states of mind similar to what is experienced with the use of LSD or meditation and spiritual practices. It helps people to understand the cause of their emotional problems and assists in healing.

Leonard Orr elaborated Rebirthing Breathworking inspired by Shri Mahavatar Babaji at his Ashram in the Himalayas. In this system inhalation and exhalation are merged with no pause in between them. It allegedly provides the opportunity to heal the birth-death cycle as well as birth trauma. This is achieved through reaching complete relaxation, a space in which no disease can live. Sondra Ray developed Liberation Breathing, which has the claim of liberating from negative thoughts and emotions, pain, mental blocks, traumatic incidents, addictions, depression and birth trauma.

Dr Judith Kravitz combined conscious breathing with psychological counselling and called her system Transformational Breath. Jacqueline Small, one of Grof's disciples, developed Integrative Breathwork, which uses music, breathing, meditative autohypnosis and symbolic artwork to release unconscious patterns.

A new breathing technique was developed in 2013 by Deanna Reiter and Troy Stende called Qi Breathing. Reiter, a student under Orr and Ray, combined breathing exercises with Qigong. This technique increases energy, reduces stress and improves health. As with all the previous researchers of breathing methods Reiter and Stende noticed that a higher quality breath results in a higher quality of life and, equally, that a richer, deeper breath promotes a richer life.

In 2020, COVID - 19 restrictions forced most of the world population to utterly disregard all the above principles and obliged us to constantly and unnaturally rebreathe our own carbon dioxide, a toxic by-product of cellular metabolism, a gas poisonous to our cells, a gas we should constantly expel to stay alive.

CHAPTER TWO

Anatomy and physiology of the respiratory system

"Everybody breathes. It's a fundamental activity that we all do, all day, every day. Our breath should be our first priority, yet it's something that we tend to ignore until it becomes a problem. Unfortunately, what most of us fail to realise is that our breathing is already a problem. The reality is that over ninety percent of us are using less than fifty percent of our breathing capacity. We are inhaling very shallowly, taking in a minimal amount of oxygen. Our exhalations are also marginal, which perpetuates a shallow inhalation. By taking in a less than ideal amount of oxygen, we are not fuelling our blood and bodies with sufficient energy. By not expelling enough carbon dioxide, we are harbouring toxins and waste in our blood streams and organs. Shallow breathing does not provide sufficient oxygen to our brain or other cells and has been linked with degenerative disease, poor quality of life and an early onset of death. Breathing is necessary for life. But what many of us don't consider is that breathing is also the quickest, easiest and most rewarding solution to deal with stress. As babies, we breathed in a full, connected rhythm through the diaphragm that allowed complete circulation in our small bodies. As we mature, that rhythm changes. For many people, a shift in breathing occurs as toddlers. By age eleven, the majority of people breathe marginally, engaging only the chest and not the solar plexus. Shallow breathing results in circulating less energy and oxygen. That likely leaves you more depressed, tired, anxious, scared or sad. Experiencing these negative emotions as they arise is not good. But what's even worse is when these

emotions are suppressed and accumulate as stored tension in the body that can later result in injury or illness. Conscious breathing helps us to feel and process emotion. It helps us bring in more oxygen to our cells and our organs so that every part of us can function better. It helps us think more clearly, digest our food and have stronger immune systems. Shallow breathing leads to physical, emotional and mental blocks. These blocks can lead to inner conflicts, imbalances, personality disorders, destructive lifestyles and disease.

Many people do not realise that there is a deeper meaning and spiritual connection of the breath. In yogic teachings, it is the breath that is our bridge between body, mind and spirit. In meditation, it is the breath that enables us to be awakened to the present moment away from our daily distractions and our busy minds." – The history of Breathing

The challenge of this chapter is to explain the main functions of the respiratory system without making this into a boring anatomy and physiology manual.

The human respiratory system is one of the most important systems of the body, we can live days without food and fluids but just 3-4 minutes without breathing. We breathe about 16,000 to 24,000 times per day and in that time, we exchange about 11,000 litres of air with the atmosphere.

The main functions of the respiratory system are supplying oxygen to the body, removing waste products such as carbon dioxide, maintaining homeostasis (acid-alkaline balance) of arterial blood and regulate heat exchange.

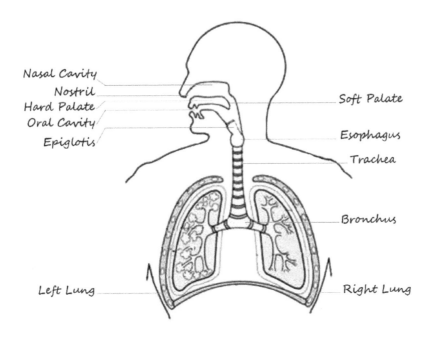

Nasal Cavity
Nostril
Hard Palate
Oral Cavity
Epiglotis

Soft Palate

Esophagus

Trachea

Bronchus

Left Lung

Right Lung

The respiratory system is a network of organs and tissues that enables respiration. It includes airways, lungs, blood vessels and the bones and muscles that contain and power the lungs. These parts work together to move oxygen throughout the body and clean out waste gases like carbon dioxide. In this process the oxygen of the atmosphere is delivered to the human body, utilised by all the tissues, transformed into carbon dioxide and other waste gases, transported back to the lungs and expelled into the atmosphere.

The respiratory system has various other functions. Besides helping inhalation and exhalation, it allows to talk and smell, warms air to match body temperature and moisturises it to the humidity level the body needs and protects the airways from harmful substances and irritants.

The vocal cords present in the larynx divide the respiratory tract into upper and lower respiratory tract. The upper respiratory tract contains structures such as the nasal cavity, the sinuses, the pharynx and the part of the larynx above the vocal cords. The lower respiratory tract starts with the part of the larynx below the vocal cords and continues with trachea, bronchi and bronchioles.

The nasal cavity has a bone roof which also form the base of the skull and a floor constituted by the palatine bones. The main job of the nose and the nasal cavity is the filtration of air. This is made possible by small hair like structures located in the nasal cavity and called cilia. Through constantly shifting in a wave-like motion, they filter dust and other irritants out of the airways. The filtration of air is also facilitated by mucus secreted by the nasal walls. This traps dust, pollens as well as other pollutants present in the atmosphere. The sinuses are hollow areas between the bones of the skull that help regulate the temperature and humidity of the inhaled air. This prevents dryness of the respiratory membranes.

The oral cavity serves as a secondary opening for the respiratory tract. The downside is that there is no filtration, no humidification and no temperature regulation through the oral cavity which is cause for several issues and the reason we should always inhale through our nostrils. In fact, human beings are the only mammals that breathe through the mouth. Other animals only do that in extremely rare circumstances and for very good reasons. The positive side is that the oral cavity has a wider opening that facilitates greater intake of air during exercise or other exceptional events. The inhaled air goes then into the pharynx which is a muscular tube that connects the oral and the nasal cavity to the larynx and the oesophagus.

When the air reaches the pharynx, it encounters two important structures: the trachea (windpipe), which lies in the front and the oesophagus in the back of our neck.

Another important element is the epiglottis, a cartilaginous structure that closes the laryngeal inlet and prevents entry of food into the trachea and consequently into the lungs. Next in the respiratory tract is the larynx, a hollow organ that allows us to talk and make sounds when air moves in and out. It is also known as the voice box or, in males, the Adam's apple. The larynx is made of many cartilages and contains the vocal cords. Its main function, beside speech, is the connection to the trachea.

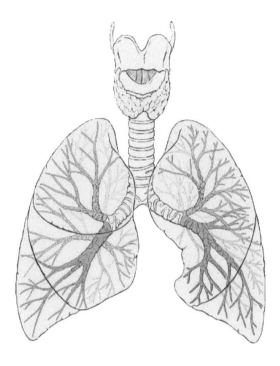

The trachea is a tube structure that connects the larynx to the bronchi. The bronchi in turn connect to the lungs. The trachea is made up of twenty 'C' shaped cartilages. These prevent the collapse of the trachea due to the fact that there is a negative pressure in the lungs and trachea during inhalation. The tracheal rings are not completely circular because the oesophagus lies behind the trachea and if these rings were circular they would compress the oesophagus during swallowing.

This could lead to choking.

The trachea brings the inhaled air into the lungs which are constituted by three lobes in the right lung and two in the left lung. The lungs are protected by the pleura, thin lubricated sacs that surround each lung lobe and separate the lungs from the chest wall. The trachea divides itself into primary bronchi, secondary bronchioles and tertiary bronchioles. The latter further divide about twenty times to form the conducting bronchioles. The conducting bronchioles then form a three to five division series of respiratory bronchioles.

The respiratory bronchioles are in turn connected to the alveoli. These are sac-like structures in which the actual gas exchange happens. The conducting bronchioles are so named because they do not facilitate gas exchange due to their thick walls. Respiratory bronchioles on the contrary have very thin walls and allow gas exchange, even though, the majority of the gas exchange happens in the alveoli due to their close proximity to the blood vessels.

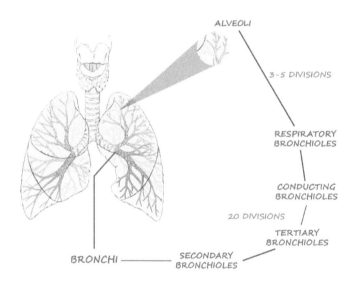

The respiratory system works in conjunction with the circulatory system to provide gas exchange. The heart receives all the deoxygenated blood from the body through the superior and the inferior vena cava. This blood has a low concentration of oxygen and is pumped to the lungs through the pulmonary arteries. In the lungs this deoxygenated blood is subjected to gas exchange which converts it into oxygenated blood. This is pumped back to the heart and to the body which then utilises the oxygen present in the blood. Once the blood is depleted of oxygen, it is pumped back to the heart to restart a new cycle. The heart pumps all the deoxygenated blood to the lungs through two main arteries the right and the left pulmonary artery. Just as we saw with the previous branching pattern in which a single bronchus divides twenty to twenty-five times before the formation of alveoli, a similar phenomenon happens with the large blood vessels that enter the lungs. These blood vessels also divide several times until the formation of small capillaries in extremely close contact with the alveoli. Capillaries are blood vessels in the alveoli walls that move oxygen and carbon dioxide. This leads to the exposure of the five litres of our blood to almost 250 to 300 million alveoli per minute through diffusion. The blood coming in, on one side of the capillary, is in its deoxygenated state and is converted into oxygenated blood on the other side. This oxygenated blood is then sent to the heart, recirculated and utilised.

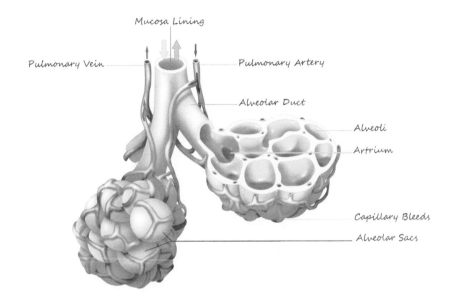

Muscles and bones help to move the inhaled air inside and outside of the lungs. The main bones and muscles in the respiratory system include the diaphragm which aids inhalation and exhalation and the ribs, bones that surround and protect lungs and heart.

In humans and most other mammals, breathing occurs also through cutaneous respiration that accounts for 1 - 2 percent of the total. It is crucial to notice, though, that our skin is our largest organ.

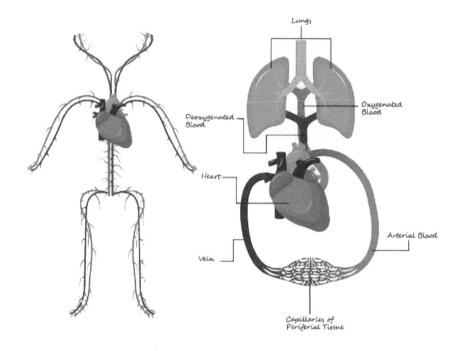

Many conditions can affect the respiratory system. Some develop due to irritants inhaled from the air, others occur as a result of disease or getting older. Conditions that can cause inflammation (swelling, irritation and pain) or otherwise affect the respiratory system include allergies, contracted through the inhalation of proteins, such as dust, mould, and pollen; asthma, a chronic disorder that causes inflammation of the airways and can make breathing difficult; infections that can lead to pneumonia (inflammation of the lungs) or bronchitis (inflammation of the bronchial tubes). Common respiratory infections include flu, COVID or cold.

Respiratory disorders include lung cancer and Chronic Obstructive Pulmonary Disease (COPD). These illnesses can harm the respiratory system's ability to deliver oxygen throughout the body and filter out waste gases. Also, lung capacity decreases with getting older.

One of the most neglected functions of the respiratory system is that, by supplying oxygen to the body and eliminating carbon dioxide, respiration also maintains the acid-alkaline balance. When this balance is disrupted, the lungs attempt to compensate. Hypoventilation or slow and shallow breathing can increase carbon dioxide levels in the blood by removing less carbon dioxide than usual. This phenomenon is amplified with mask wearing. On the contrary, hyperventilation or rapid and deep breathing can cause more carbon dioxide to be eliminated.

Chemoreceptors react to the cerebral spinal fluid pH, impacted by blood pH and acts upon the respiratory centre in the brain to correct the imbalance. If the pH is low (acidosis), the chemoreceptors stimulate the respiratory centre to increase the respiratory rate, in an effort to normalise it. On the contrary, if the pH is high (alkalosis), the chemoreceptors will stimulate the respiratory centre to decrease the respiratory rate. Peripheral receptors in the aorta and carotid bodies also respond to these changes in blood pH, and stimulate the respiratory centre. Although we normally think of the lungs as being critical in oxygenating the cells of the body, the elimination of carbon dioxide is vital to pH regulation. Blood pH value should remain between 7.35 and 7.45. When the pH is within this range, along with normal oxygen levels, the respiratory system is functioning at its best, keeping our tissues well oxygenated and removing the waste products of the cells adequately.

Mask wearing disrupts this process completely and causes a rampant rise in acidosis due to shallow breathing and lack of proper removal of carbon dioxide. Ultimately the cells of our body suffocate in our own waste products. Cancer cells thrive in acidity (low pH), but not in alkalinity (high pH). This is one of the many ways mask wearing is going to kill you.

CHAPTER THREE

Pranayama, sleeping patterns and other stories

"When the breath is unsteady, all is unsteady; when the breath is still; all is still. Control the breath carefully. Inhalation gives strength and a controlled body; retention gives steadiness of mind and longevity; exhalation purifies body and spirit." – Goraksasathakam

Before discussing pranayama, it is necessary to define what prana is. The only way I can possibly do this, in simple terms, is through telling my mother's story. In the beginning of this account, she was a very healthy person, coming from a patriarchal, 'Mediterranean diet' family. I am talking about the proper Mediterranean diet of the forties and fifties in the south of Italy in which everyone would grow their own vegetables, organic was the only possible option, breakfast consisted of climbing a tree and eating whichever fruit was in season at that time of the year, bread was made with home grown grains and baked once a week in the village wood burning oven. Meat intake was 750 grams on Thursday, shared by thirteen people, and 1.5 kilos on Sundays, consumed with the same number of family members. My mother has been growing fruit and vegetables since and visits to doctors and dentists were a very rare event.

All of this changed when my sister, a qualified doctor, gave her for Christmas a brand-new microwave oven. From then on, my mother completely disregarded her six-ring gas hob. Happy with her new toy, especially because the gift was coming from a respected clinician, there was no meal or food that would not end up some way or another in her microwave. From homemade tomato sauce to reheated Lavazza coffee.

At first, she just gained weight, it seemed that food was no longer nourishing her and she had cravings for sugar and cakes and anything that would provide her with a surplus of calories.

Then things went worse and a few months down the line, she was diagnosed with breast, stomach and uterus cancer. She is still alive and well after operations, radiotherapy, chemotherapy and whatever else allopathic medicine prescribed her to do or take.

Prana is the life energy that was contained in my mother's food before the microwave would completely kill it. Of course, you may decide that if you cannot perceive something, then, it is not real. It would be the same as saying that electricity does not exist because you cannot see it and expect not to get electrocuted when you put your wet fingers on a live wire. Prana is the 'negative ions' feeling that you get after a storm, is the perception of being energised after a walk on a pristine and unaltered tropical beach. The fact that you may not believe in it does not stop it doing its vital job.

The core issue is that despite living in the twenty-first century where the scientific frontier has expanded into the study of Quantum Physics, the Unified field, the Holographic principle, Epigenetic, the electromagnetic nature of the human body and the Terrain view, the 'science' we follow is an outdated and invalid eightieth century's vision of the Universe. This despite the fact that Newton admitted on his death bed to have proposed an incomplete scientific truth devoid of the existence of the God in which he believed. He also, in secret, performed several alchemical experiments. Ultimately, Newton hoped his scientific writings would lead people to think about and believe in God rather than deviate in a mere mechanistic outlook of physics.

Similarly, Louis Pasteur, another modern-day idol, confessed to gross scientific misconduct and fraud. Pasteur declared in his diary to have faked many aspects of his research studies on human beings and test animals in order to prove viral transmission and to have pursued a never proved, to this day, Germ theory. He also stated, in the last days of his life that

Claude Bernard's Terrain view was superior to his own and deemed that as the correct path to follow. Modern 'science' is in total denial of all the above and stubbornly behaves as an extinct Diplodocus.

I do not even wish to debate what Florence Nightingale, another Terrain Theory proposer would have said of the way we deal with COVID, she is probably busy turning in her grave as I write. It is my opinion that quantum physics, yoga, pranayama and other spiritual traditions share several common notions. Our 37.2 trillion of cells constitute a miniature biome that needs to work in unison and harmony within a larger ecosystem in order for us to be healthy. Even a minimal disruption in one organ will affect all the others and cause the whole house of cards to collapse.

Mechanistic reductionism in relation to physical reality does not work in our complex universe. The human body is not simply a machine that we can dissemble and put back together as we do with our car parts. In the organ transplant field there is a plethora of stories of human recipients assuming the donor's psychological traits. This is somehow acceptable when the phenomena are limited to peanut butter cravings or having a newly born artistic ability, but what implications does this bring when the donors were Chinese Falun Gong practitioners strapped to a bed and still alive whilst their organs were illegally harvested?

Let's not dive in this any further and go back to pranayama for the time being. Every human being absorbs prana via the respiratory system including cutaneous respiration which accounts for 1 - 2% of the total through the biggest organ, the skin, and by way of food consumption.

Modern human beings are unhealthier than previous generations, when food never came from tins, cans, tetra pack and McDonald's. Add to this air pollution, stress and mask wearing and there you have it: the immune system cannot cope with all of this and sickness begins.

Pranayama is the practice of breath regulation and one of the eight pillars of yoga. In Sanskrit, "prana" means life energy and "yama" means control. The practice of pranayama involves breathing exercises. The benefits of pranayama have been extensively researched.

According to scientific studies, pranayama may benefit human health in many ways. For example, it decreases stress and mood and anxiety disorders.

It has been estimated that about 28% of Europeans suffer from those conditions during their life. Negative thinking and emotional and behavioural avoidance are some of the negative effects experienced and those factors lead to higher health care utilisation, less work productivity, social and economic dysfunctions and lower quality of life. Major depression increases the risk of suicide and death from other conditions such as coronary artery disease and diabetes.

Cognitive behavioural therapy and pharmacology improve acute symptoms but the benefits for patients are shown to be moderate and normally those treatments do not improve chronic or treatment resistant instances.

Just few days ago it has been determined that depression is not due to chemical imbalance and medication cannot actually sort the issue. Yoga in general and pranayama in particular are utilised as ancillary or alternative methods because it has been indicated that such an approach helps to alleviate psychological distress and the associated negative thinking and emotional and behavioural issues. Yoga and pranayama could also be considered as interventions due to their acceptability by the general public, especially those individuals that do not seek treatment or easily drop out of their established therapy.

On the biochemical and neurophysiological level there is evidence that yoga and pranayama practice can cause modifications in many biological processes that produce mood alteration and depression.

For example, specific exercises increase the internal release of dopamine, decrease the dysregulation of certain endocrine glands such as hypothalamus, pituitary and adrenals that generate stress response and reduce levels of plasma cortisol.

In practice, pranayama reduces perceived stress levels, calms the nervous system and improves stress response.

Scientific studies invariably determine that individuals who practice pranayama experience less anxiety before taking a test. The authors of the studies link this effect to the increased oxygen intake during the exercises. As explained many times so far, oxygen is energy for the human body's vital organs and this includes brain and nerves. In conclusion, yoga and pranayama improve stress, depression and anxiety disorders and mask wearing just cause the opposite.

The stress-relieving effects of pranayama may also help you sleep. And this opens to an unimaginable amount of health benefits. In clinical studies, a technique known as Bhramari pranayama is shown to slow down breathing and heart rate when practiced for at least five minutes. This helps calm the body and prepare it for sleep.

According to another study pranayama also improves sleep quality in people with obstructive sleep apnoea. Additionally, the study found that practicing pranayama decreases snoring and daytime sleepiness, suggesting benefits for better quality rest. If you think that the above are minor and negligible benefits, I really invite you to think again.

Recently I attended two dementia conferences that proved strict correlations between sleeping patterns and the insurgence and prevention of various cognitive disorders and Alzheimer's disease.

A presentation in particular: "Understanding how sleep and circadian rhythms contribute to brain function" by Professor Derk-Jan Dijk, Professor of Sleep and Physiology, Director at Surrey Sleep Research Centre, made the penny drop big time. So, what causes Alzheimer's disease? In our brains billions of specialised cells called neurons process and transmit information through electrical and chemical signals. Messages are continuously sent to different parts of the brain, and from the brain to the body. Alzheimer's disease causes a breakdown in communication between neurons and this causes loss of function and cell death. As a direct consequence of the decrease of cell numbers, large areas in the brain begin to shrink. During the final stage brain atrophy is widespread with significant loss of brain volume.

According to the USA National Institute of Ageing, Alzheimer's is caused by Amyloid Plaques, Tau and Neurofibrillary Tangles. In the first instance, the beta-amyloid protein formed from the breakdown of a larger protein (amyloid precursor protein) is involved in the insurgence of Alzheimer's. It comes in several different molecular forms and accumulates between neurons.

The beta-iamyloid 42 is especially harmful. In Alzheimer's, abnormal levels of this naturally occurring protein clump together to form plaques that collect between neurons and disrupt cell function. Research is ongoing to better understand how, and at what stage of the disease, the various forms of beta-amyloid influence Alzheimer's.

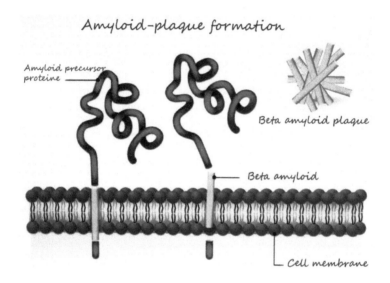

Amyloid-plaque formation

Amyloid precursor proteine

Beta amyloid plaque

Beta amyloid

Cell membrane

In the second case, neurofibrillary tangles are abnormal accumulations of proteins called tau that collect inside neurons. Neurons, are partially supported internally by structures called microtubules Their function is to facilitate the passage of nutrients and molecules from the cell body to the axon and dendrites. In healthy neurons, Tau is normally bonded to the microtubules and stabilises them. In Alzheimer's disease, on the contrary, abnormal chemical changes cause tau to separate from microtubules and attach to other tau molecules, forming threads that eventually join to form stacks. These block the neuron's transport system harming the synaptic communication between neurons.

Alzheimer's-related brain changes may result from a complex interplay among abnormal tau and beta-amyloid proteins and several other factors. As follows, I will explain how sleep protects against Alzheimer's insurgence.

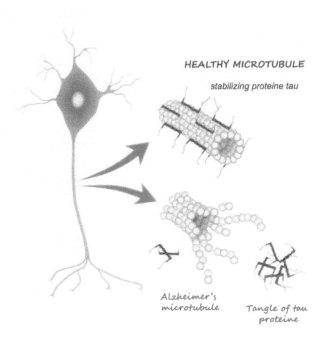

HEALTHY MICROTUBULE

stabilizing proteine tau

Alzheimer's microtubule

Tangle of tau proteine

There is a key relationship between sleep and loss of cognitive functions. It is not clear whether poor sleep causes or worsens Alzheimer's or if Alzheimer's leads to poor sleep. Both of these theories could be true, and the relationship could be circular.

During deep sleep, our brains are working hard to wash away the waste products that increase the risk for Alzheimer's disease.

This process is controlled by our glymphatic system, a waste clearance network of our central nervous system that while we are sleeping clears proteins, toxins, and other debris.

Poor sleep makes the glymphatic system less efficient and the accumulation of toxic substances could lead to inflammation and degeneration of the neurons that over time leads to Alzheimer's.

Several studies suggest that deep sleep - when body temperature drops and the brain begins to produce slow, rhythmic electrical waves, when dreams are rare and the brain follows a slow, steady beat – can help reduce levels of beta-amyloid and tau.

Without adequate sleep, our brain cannot effectively wash away these precursor proteins.

Matthew Walker, a professor of neuroscience and psychology at the University of California suggests that it is now possible to look into the future and accurately estimate how much beta-amyloid it is going to be accumulated over the next years, simply on the basis of the present quality of someone's sleep.

Walker's team studied thirty-two people in their seventies who had taken part in a sleep study that looked for the slow electrical waves that signal deep sleep. The scientists used brain scans to monitor levels of beta-amyloid in each participant for up to six years. The results, published in the journal 'Current Biology', showed that people who got less deep sleep had more beta-amyloid.

Scientists have some ideas about why deep sleep seems to be able to reduce both beta-amyloid and tau.

In 2013, a landmark study of mice found that their brains switched on a sort of dishwasher during sleep and beta amyloid plaques and tau stacks were removed more rapidly from their brains when asleep versus when they were awake.

In 2019, Sarah Lewis led a team that showed how this dishwasher works in people. There are waves of fluid flowing into the brain during sleep and each wave of fluid is preceded by a large, slow electrical wave. Now scientists are looking for ways to induce the slow waves that signal deep sleep. In people, there is some evidence that rhythmic sounds can increase slow waves. Deep sleep can also be achieved by treating sleep disorders.

Obstructive sleep apnoea is most common in older people and people with obesity. Apnoea induces a higher risk of cognitive decline because it may cause damage to the brain due to changes of levels of oxygen and carbon dioxide in the blood and incidentally, wearing masks provokes the very same phenomenon. Sleep apnoea may also change the flow of blood to the brain. These patients seem to have a change in their ability to clear proteins or waste products from their brain. After patients had been treated successfully for apnoea the results were increase in deep sleep, more beta-amyloid cleared and less produced in the brain.

Light sleep disorders, often called rapid eye movement sleep behaviour disorder (RBD) are a very early indicator of Alzheimer's, particularly in older men.

Sleep-wake cycle disorders are another concern when it comes to dementia and Alzheimer's.

A circadian rhythm or circadian cycle is a natural, internal process that regulates the sleep–wake cycle. When this cycle is altered unusual and disruptive sleep patterns occur.

Any disruptions in sleeping patterns may increase risks of Alzheimer's and dementia or may even be an early sign of these diseases.

Adequate sleep is about both quantity and quality. A common misconception is that as people age, they need less sleep. Sleep quantity must be and has to be between seven and eight hours on a regular basis and it has to be consecutive sleeping.

Harvard Medical School found a 36% increased risk of cognitive decline in women who reported sleeping six or fewer hours a night and a 35% increased risk in those who said they slept longer than eight hours.

Mentally, poor sleep can lead to anxiety, depression, poor memory, and degenerative diseases like Alzheimer's and dementia. This can occur especially if we have an underlying sleep disorder and/or don't sleep long enough.

Adequate sleep is also defined by the stages of sleep. The stages of sleep are all essential for promoting good health. Often REM stages of sleep are the first to get 'skipped' during sleep issues or disorders.

Poor sleep can result in trouble managing weight, diabetes and thyroid dysfunction due to hormone dysregulation. These are also factors in the insurgence of Alzheimer's. It's in the deeper stages of sleep when our hormones reset.

When our stress levels increase, sleep is often affected. Various stressors can create sleep disruptions.

The best way to reduce stress or to be able to handle stressful situations is to be adequately rested. Regular sleep regimes, eating schedules and diets, exercise, and ensuring exposure to bright light in the morning are all ways that you can improve your sleep quality.

Some drug treatments for poor sleep, such as benzodiazepines, have been linked to an increased risk of dementia.

On the contrary, melatonin ($C_{13}H_{16}N_2O_2$), a hormone naturally produced by the pineal gland during sleep is important in maintaining regular sleep-wake cycles and improves sleep quality in people with Alzheimer's and Parkinson's disease. Furthermore, Melatonin does not present any risk of dementia or cognitive function.

In a nutshell, and in a sort of domino effect, pranayama helps your sleep, resolves obstructive sleep apnoea and produces better quality rest. This removes some of the main causes of the insurgence of dementia and other degenerative cognitive illnesses. In the final stage of writing this book I have learnt that the amyloid plaque and Tau stack theory of causation for Alzheimer's disease has been questioned as probably incorrect and pursued only to promote the use of specific medication.

On the contrary, everything that has been described above in relation to the importance of sleeping, removing toxins and the related aid provided by the millenary yoga and pranayama tradition remains the best course of action to counteract cognitive degeneration. It is useful to note that this discipline encompasses every aspect of human activity, from diet, ethics, mental and emotional self-regulation.

In fact, pranayama improves mental awareness. Individuals who practices it display higher levels of mindfulness and emotional regulation than those who do not. This is associated with the calming effect of pranayama, which supports the ability to be more mindful. Pranayama helps remove carbon dioxide and raises oxygen concentration, which fuels brain cells. This may contribute to mindfulness by improving focus and concentration.

Furthermore, pranayama has a substantial effect on high blood pressure, or hypertension. This can also increase the risk of some potentially serious health conditions like heart disease and stroke. Stress is a major risk factor for high blood pressure. Pranayama can help minimise this danger by promoting relaxation.

In a 2014 study, participants with mild hypertension received antihypertensive drugs for six weeks. Half the participants also received pranayama training for 6 weeks. By the end of the study, the latter group experienced a greater reduction in blood pressure.

This effect, according to the study authors, is likely due to the mindful breathing of pranayama. Concentration on breathing can help calm your nervous system, this consequently may reduce your stress response and the risk of hypertension.

Pranayama also improves lung functions and strengthen the respiratory organs through the slow, and forceful breathing of the exercises.

A 2019 study determined that six weeks of practicing pranayama for one hour daily could have a significant effect on lung functions. The practice improves multiple parameters according to pulmonary test results.

Pranayama may be useful in many respiratory system disorders including asthma, allergic bronchitis and can be utilised to improve recovery in pneumonia and tuberculosis.

In addition to benefiting your lungs, pranayama may also enhance your brain function and enhances cognitive performances. A 2013 study found that twelve weeks of pranayama improved memory, cognitive flexibility, reasoning skills and enhanced the perception of own level of stress and reaction time. Additionally, the study found that fast pranayama was associated with better auditory memory and sensory-motor performance. According to the researchers, these benefits are, once more, due to the stress-lowering effects of pranayama and the increased oxygen uptake, which energises brain cells.

Finally, there is evidence that yogic breathing, or pranayama, could decrease cravings in people who are trying to quit smoking. In a 2012 study, just 10 minutes of yogic breathing caused a short-term reduction in cigarette cravings. A more recent study found, similarly, that mindfulness-based yoga breathing decreases the negative effects associated with smoking withdrawal.

How does 'surgical mask wearing' fit with all the above? The answer is quite plain and simple. It does not. It just aggravates and disrupts natural biological functions and wherever pranayama brings benefits, described here in detail, mask wearing produces only opposite and detrimental effects.

We seem to easily forget that we are part of a natural ecosystem in which every structure in our body is strictly connected with all the others and tampering with one aspect of our physiological functioning affects our wellbeing in ways that we rarely consider. I have been closely observing patients sleeping with their mask on. The damage they provoke to their health is unimaginable.

Humans are not supposed to wear masks because the human body was simply not designed to wear them. It is simply not healthy, no matter what the government or large corporations say, to block one's breathing passages with fabric or plastic. There is no scientific evidence to show that wearing a mask does anything beneficial. In fact, the latest research shows that wearing a mask does pretty much nothing besides damage.

Why, then, are many politicians, pharmaceutical companies, and media still pushing them? The answer is anyone's guess.

In the quote at the start of this chapter, Goraksasathakam states that exhalation purifies body and spirit. None of that can happen when someone traps and rebreathes their own carbon dioxide. Would you eat or drink the waste products coming from your body? Rebreathing them does not produce any better outcome.

In the next chapters we will explore in detail the damage triggered by mask wearing throughout the human life span and on all levels: physical, emotional, psychological social, sociological and spiritual.

CHAPTER FOUR

Masks and peer reviewed articles

"Deep breathing brings deep thinking and shallow breathing brings shallow thinking." – Elsie Lincoln Benedict

A recent research study of May 2022, "Inhaled CO_2 concentration while wearing face masks: a pilot study using capnography" from Ferrara (Italy) reported the following conclusions:

"Shortly after wearing surgical masks, the inhaled CO_2 approached the highest acceptable exposure threshold recommended for workers, while concerningly high concentrations were recorded in virtually all individuals when wearing FFP2 masks. The CO_2 concentration was significantly higher among minors and subjects with high respiratory rate."

The study determined that wearing a face mask result in exposure to dangerous concentrations of carbon dioxide even when the mask is worn for just five minutes and just sitting still. CO_2 concentration exceeded the danger zone of 5,000 ppm (part per million) in 40% of cases. Whilst wearing FFP2 masks, it exceeded it in 99% of cases.

The study used a technique called capnography to take the measurements of CO_2 in inhaled air over the course of five minutes, following a ten minute period of rest, with participants seated, silent and breathing only through the nose. A doctor took measurements at minutes three, four and five, with an average of the three measurements being used in the analysis.

The study found that the mean CO_2 concentration of inhaled air without masks was 458 ppm. While wearing a surgical mask, the mean CO_2 was over 10 times higher at 4,965 ppm, exceeding 5,000 ppm in 40.2% of the measurements. While wearing an FFP2 mask, the average CO_2 was nearly double again at 9,396 ppm, with 99.0% of participants showing values higher than 5,000 ppm.

Among children under eighteen, the mean CO_2 concentration while wearing a surgical mask was well above the safe limit at 6,439 ppm; for a FFP2 mask it was nearly double again at 12,847 ppm. The researchers found that breaths per minute only had to increase by three, from fifteen to eighteen, for the mean concentration to reach 5,271 ppm in a surgical mask and breach the safe limit.

While the findings are clearly concerning enough, the researchers note that "the experimental conditions, with participants at complete rest and in a constantly ventilated room, were far from those experienced by workers and students during a typical day, normally spent in rooms shared with other people or doing some degree of physical activity".

In such conditions the CO_2 concentration of inhaled air is likely to be considerably higher.

In a mental health setting, an average day at work is very rarely about sitting in the office and breathing slowly and calmly, it rather consists in running around corridors, going up and down staircases, being involved in PMVA (Prevention and Managing of Violence and Aggression) interventions, restrains and various other straining activities. And the above does not last only five minutes but it is rather endured for twelve to fourteen hours, day in and day out.

While the Italian study did not focus on the reduction in blood oxygen saturation during the five minutes of observation of a person at rest, the authors note that another research on fifty-three surgeons wearing masks for an extended period of time found that blood oxygen saturation decreased noticeably (Preliminary report on surgical mask induced deoxygenation during major surgery - PubMed - nih.gov).

They added that exposure to CO_2 in inhaled air at concentrations exceeding 5,000 ppm for long periods is 'considered unacceptable for the workers, and is forbidden in several countries, because it frequently causes signs and symptoms such as headache, nausea, drowsiness, rhinitis and reduced cognitive performance.'

I would add dry mouth and harbouring of bacteria that lead to oral problems and periodontitis.

The authors note that this is the first study to assess properly the CO_2 concentration of inhaled air while wearing a face mask. Two earlier studies were small and did not adequately remove water vapour. A third and recent one, was retracted for, among other concerns, not using a capnograph to distinguish between inhaled and exhaled air. The above study addresses these problems.

On the opposite side of the spectrum there is the Bangladesh study of December 2021 that claims that surgical masks are 'safe and effective' (nowadays the most abused three words), and limit the spread of infections.

This cluster Randomised Control Trial (RCT) was based on dubious statistics data, began with illogical suppositions, and failed to consider the lethal risks of masks. This is the only study that claims that "masks slow the spread of contagious respiratory diseases" and attempts to prove that "mask mandates (or strategies like handing out masks at churches and other public events), could save thousands of lives each day globally."

In reality, this study excludes data that could prove or disprove those very claims, it is in violation of research ethics and aims to hide the harms of masks, which are far more common and serious than portrayed by governments and the media. The pre-analysis plan for the study states that it will measure "hospitalisations and mortality," but these measures are completely absent from the study results. This is a flagrant breach of research ethics, and it obscures the only data that can objectively prove whether masks save or cost lives. The primary reason for pre-analysis plans "is to avoid many of the issues associated with data mining by setting out in advance the specifications that will be run and with which variables."

To accurately measure the impact of masking or any other medical intervention on death, one has to measure actual deaths—not some other variable. This is because measuring whether masks prevent COVID-19 infections, a focal point of the Bangladesh study, does not measure how many people died from COVID-19 or ascertain any of the lethal risks of masks identified in medical journals, such as: cardio-pulmonary events, elevated CO_2 inhalation which can impair high-level brain functions and lead to fatal mistakes, social isolation which can lead to drug abuse and suicide, heat, humidity, and other discomforts of wearing a mask, which can cause increased error rates and response times in situations where mental sharpness is vital to safety.

Only RCTs that measure deaths can capture the net effects of all such factors. That's why medical journals call "all-cause mortality" in RCTs 'the most important outcome'.

Simply measuring all the deaths among people who receive or do not receive a treatment proves whether this saves more lives than it takes.

Beyond excluding the death data, the authors engaged in other actions that reflect poor integrity. The worst is meddling with findings.

For example, the study's "primary outcome," was a positive blood test for COVID-19 antibodies. This found that less than 1% of the participants caught COVID-19, 0.68% in villages where people were pressured to wear masks and 0.76% in villages that were not. This is a total difference of 0.08 percentage points in a study of more than 300,000 people which is, obviously, not statistically relevant.

Their analysis tested only 3% (10,790 of 342,126) of the participants. This sample may not reflect the other 97% for several reasons. For example the study didn't attempt to test people for COVID-19 unless the "owner of the household's primary phone" admitted that a member of their household had symptoms like a fever, sore throat, fatigue, and headache; 60% of the people who reportedly had symptoms did not submit to a

COVID-19 test; the analysis assumes that the following "mask promotion interventions" had no effect on the objectivity or willingness of participants to accurately report symptoms: making them watch "a brief video of notable public figures discussing why, how, and when to wear a mask"; sending them "twice-weekly text message reminders about the importance of mask-wearing"; asking them to make "a verbal commitment to be a mask-wearing household"; asking "to place signage on doors that declares they are a mask-wearing household"; giving a "monetary incentive" of 190 US dollars to "the village leader" if at least 75% of the village adults wore masks.

Furthermore their study engages in the dishonest practice of data dredging by featuring results that were not included in their pre-analysis plan, like "imputing symptomatic-seroprevalence for missing blood draws." This allows them to transform statistically insignificant results into significant ones.

In conclusion, diplodocus science loves to continuously cite the faulty Bangladesh study which was published in Science despite the efforts of many scientists in asking for its withdrawal. The Italian study, which is rigorously and scientifically set up and whose findings are cautionary advocated is not yet peer reviewed because it does not serve the present propaganda.

Recently, the UK government has removed mask mandates in public venues. Paradoxically, we experience the return to a mask-free society everywhere but in Universities, the NHS and health allied venues. Students, staff and visitors are still coerced to wear masks in some universities, all hospitals, health centres, GP practices and most pharmacies, dentists and opticians consulting rooms.

Locations that should be run by evidence-based practice, are callously persisting with unscientific and damaging mass masking. The endurance of this phenomenon in medical environments represents the triumph of culture over science. Do not be fooled into believing that anyone in there is "following the science".

The truth, in synthesis, is that governments endorsed mask mandates based on the false assumption that COVID-19 is mainly transmitted by large droplets that are bigger than the pore sizes of most masks and only remain airborne for a few seconds.

In reality, COVID-19 is mainly spread by microscopic aerosols that remain airborne for days, easily penetrate common masks, and travel freely through gaps around their edges.

Furthermore, scientific studies have found inconsistent benefits from N95 masks in healthcare settings and no statistically significant benefits from any type of mask in community settings. Most governments select and distort low-quality and unrealistic studies to support the claim that masks have effects on the spread of COVID.

By now it is a proven fact that masks, especially the N95 type, cause headaches, oral problems, difficulty breathing, increased cardio-pulmonary stress and many emotional, social and psychological disorders. In this chapter we determined that the average CO_2 concentrations inhaled by people wearing masks are far above what many governments permit for indoor settings, and this may impair certain high-level brain functions like initiative, strategic thinking, and complex decision-making.

In the following one we explore in detail the several physical consequences on our health and body homeostasis.

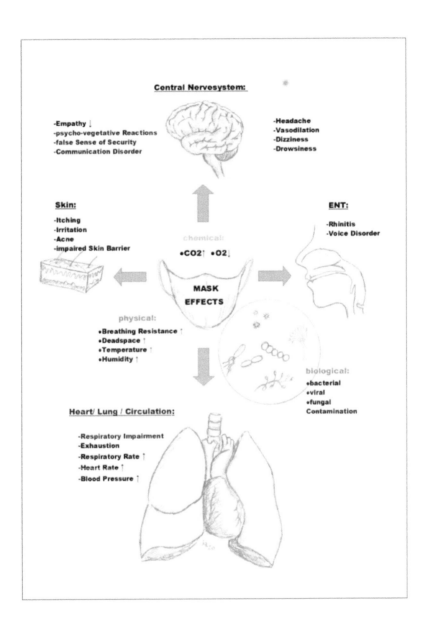

Central Nervesystem:

-Empathy ↓
-psycho-vegetative Reactions
-false Sense of Security
-Communication Disorder

-Headache
-Vasodilation
-Dizziness
-Drowsiness

Skin:

-Itching
-Irritation
-Acne
-impaired Skin Barrier

ENT:

-Rhinitis
-Voice Disorder

chemical:

• CO_2↑ • O_2↓

MASK EFFECTS

physical:

• Breathing Resistance ↑
• Deadspace ↑
• Temperature ↑
• Humidity ↑

biological:

• bacterial
• viral
• fungal
Contamination

Heart/ Lung / Circulation:

-Respiratory Impairment
-Exhaustion
-Respiratory Rate ↑
-Heart Rate ↑
-Blood Pressure ↑

CHAPTER FIVE

Masks: physical harm

"All chronic pain, suffering, and diseases are caused by a lack of oxygen at the cell level." – Dr Arthur C. Guyton

In this chapter the focus is on the physical harm caused by mask wearing. In the references, the reader can access about two hundred studies that confirm this assumption. Unfortunately, this portion of the book contains tedious but necessary data, listed in order to prove that every affirmation is based on scientific evidence. Feel free to skip through the various parts and utilise what is relevant for you.

We will start exploring the initial response to the pandemic by the World Health Organisation (WHO).

On one side, the WHO tried to stop the spread of false information in regard to anyone claiming that 'wearing a face mask can make the wearer sick' and on the other hand, in June 2020, published an 'interim guidance' stating exactly what 'disinformation sources' have been saying since the beginning of the enforcement of mask mandates.

According to the above-mentioned guidance, "The likely disadvantages of the use of masks by healthy people in the general public include: potential increased risk of self-contamination due to the manipulation of a face mask and subsequently touching eyes with contaminated hands; potential self-contamination that can occur if non-medical masks are not changed when wet or soiled. This can create favourable conditions for microorganism to amplify; potential headache and/or breathing difficulties, depending on type of mask used; a false sense of security, leading to potentially lower adherence to other critical preventive measures such as physical distancing and hand hygiene."

Scientific studies prove, beyond any doubt, that those are indeed confirmed risks and list many other factors and diseases in which masks are a definitive health hazard, even conducive to the possible death of the wearer.

For example, a cross sectional study among 343 healthcare professionals *Adverse Effects of Prolonged Mask Use among Healthcare Professionals during COVID-19*, primarily located in New York City, who worked in the hospital during the COVID-19 pandemic completed an anonymous survey consisting of twenty-one questions regarding adverse effects of PPE, medical history, and demographics. The results determined that 314 respondents reported adverse effects from prolonged mask use with headaches being the most common complaint (245) followed by skin breakdown (175) and acne (182). Impaired cognition was reported in 81 individuals. Previous history of headaches (98), skin sensitivity (164), and acne (121) were found in some cases. Some individuals experienced resolved side effects once masks were removed, while others required physical or medical intervention. In conclusion, prolonged use of N95 and surgical masks by healthcare professionals during COVID-19 has caused adverse effects such as headaches, rash, acne, skin breakdown, and impaired cognition in the majority of those surveyed.

Furthermore, many so called 'experts' seem to be unaware or purposely ignore that COVID propagates through aerosols, not droplets. Sometimes they do not even understand the difference between the two terms, as shown in the following sentence written on social media by the ubiquitous and iniquitous "independent third-party" fact checkers, where they treat these words as synonyms: "The purpose of these masks is to reduce contact with infectious droplets (aerosols), which can be generated by someone who coughs or sneezes, and thereby minimise the risk of infection transmission."

Finally, a German study published on MDPI (Multidisciplinary Digital Publishing Institute) in April 2021 analysed forty-four scientific research studies and sixty - five publications in order to list all the proven physical, sociological and psychological adverse effects of wearing masks "described because of their consistent, recurrent and uniform presentation from different disciplines as a Mask-Induced Exhaustion Syndrome (MIES)." This study is titled "Is a Mask That Covers the Mouth and Nose Free from Undesirable Side Effects in Everyday Use and Free of Potential Hazards?" I consider this as one of the most meticulous and conclusive research on the subject and I used the related findings as a major structure for this and the following chapters. The authors state:

"The literature review confirms that relevant, undesired medical, organ and organ system-related phenomena accompanied by wearing masks occur in the fields of internal medicine (at least 11 publications). The list covers neurology (seven publications), psychology (more than 10 publications), psychiatry (three publications), gynaecology (three publications), dermatology (at least 10 publications), ENT medicine (four publications), dentistry (one publication), sports medicine (four publications), sociology (more than five publications), occupational medicine (more than fourteen publications), microbiology (at least four publications), epidemiology (more than sixteen publications), and paediatrics (four publications) as well as environmental medicine (four publications)."

As follows a non-exhaustive list of physical damage and adverse reactions proven by this and other hundreds of scientific investigations on this topic:

- Headache

- Increase in dead space volume

- Increase in breathing resistance and restriction of airflow

- Increase in blood carbon dioxide (Hypercapnia)

- Decrease in blood oxygen saturation (Hypoxia and hypoxemia)

- Decrease in cardiopulmonary capacity

- Overall perceived fatigue and exhaustion

- Increase in heart rate

- Increase in respiratory rate and irregular pulse (arrhythmia)

- Difficulty breathing and shortness of breath (dyspnoea)

- Dizziness

- Feeling of dampness and heat

- Drowsiness

- Decreased ability to concentrate

- Decreased ability to think

- Decrease in empathy perception

- Impaired skin barrier function with acne, itching and skin lesions

- Increased risk of falls in the elderly

- Increase risk of insurgence of obesity

- Overall perceived fatigue and exhaustion

The possible side effects and dangers of masks described in the following studies are based on different types of masks. These include surgical mask and N95/N99 (FFP2 and FFP3 UK equivalent) that are commonly used in everyday life, but also community fabric masks.

In the case of N95/N99, the N stands for National Institute for Occupational Safety and Health of the United States (NIOSH), and 95/99 indicates the 95 or 99 per cent filtering capacity for fine particles up to at least 0.3 μm.

Headaches

A range of studies show that surgical and N95 masks induce headaches in some people.

In 2009, the "American Journal of Infection Control" published the results of a small RCT (Randomised Control Trial) on surgical masks involving thirty-two healthcare workers for seventy-seven consecutive days. It found that workers assigned to wear masks "were significantly more likely to experience headache" than the mask-less group. On average, the daily headache rate for non-mask wearing workers was 1.3%, while it was 4.9% for mask wearers, a 3.8-fold increase.

Similarly, a study published in 2019 by the journal "BMC Infectious Diseases" found that 6% of hospital workers who wore a surgical mask for one shift reported a headache.

Due to the fact that N95 masks have enhanced filters and tighter fits on the mouth than surgical masks, they restrict breathing greatly, cause higher facial pressure, and are more uncomfortable. Consequently, a study published in 2006 by the journal "Acta Neurologica Scandinavica" found that 37.3% of 212 frontline healthcare workers in a Chinese hospital "reported headaches when they wore the N95 face mask." Among these workers who experienced headaches, 62.7% "had no pre-existing headaches."

Similarly, a study published in 2020 by the journal "Headache" evaluated 158 frontline healthcare workers in a Singapore hospital, early during the COVID-19 pandemic, and found that 81.0% of them developed headaches when wearing personal protective equipment, which included N95 masks and eye protection. Among the workers who had a pre-existing problem with headaches, 91.3% "agreed" or "strongly agreed" that "the increased PPE usage had affected the control of their background headaches, which affected their level of work performance". Among the workers who experienced headaches 53.1% thought that "the N95 mask was the likely cause of a headache", 81.3% developed a headache within sixty minutes of putting on the mask, 88% had a "headache resolved spontaneously" within thirty minutes of taking off the mask.

In another study on N95 masks, initial headaches were experienced by up to 82% of 158 twenty one to thirty five year old mask wearers with one third (34%) experiencing headaches up to four times daily. Participants wore the mask for 18.3 days over a thirty day period with a mean of 5.9 hours per day, which again is far from the average working shift of 12-14 hours in care settings.

Significantly increased headache could be observed not only for N95 but also for surgical masks in participants of another observational study of health care workers.

In another study, the researchers classified 306 users with an average age of 43 years and wearing different types of masks, of whom 51% had an initial headache as a specific symptom related exclusively to increased surgical and N95 mask use (1 to 4 hours).

Researchers from Singapore were able to demonstrate in a trial involving 154 healthy N95 mask wearers working in care a significant increase in mask-induced blood carbon dioxide levels and a measurably greater vasodilatation with an increase in cerebral artery flow in the cerebra media. This was associated with headaches in the trial group.

According to the researchers, the aforementioned changes also contribute to headaches during the prolonged use of masks with a shift towards hypoxia and hypercapnia. Furthermore, stress and mechanical factors such as the irritation of cervical nerves in the neck and head area caused by the tight mask straps pressuring the nerve strands also contribute to headaches.

In the analysis of the primary studies, it was possible to detect an association between the N95 mask and headaches with all the related neurological consequences that this may lead to. In six out of 10 studies, the significant headache appeared in conjunction with the N95 mask (60% of all studies).

Dead space, breathing difficulties and Carbon dioxide

According to the scientific data, mask wearers as a whole show a conspicuous frequency of "typical, measurable, physiological changes associated with masks".

In recent studies, measurements of the gas content for oxygen and carbon dioxide under a mask showed a lower oxygen availability, even at rest, than without a mask.

Dead space represents the volume of ventilated air that does not participate in gas exchange. The anatomical dead space is represented by the volume of air that fills the areas of respiration made up by the nose, trachea, and bronchi. Masks expand the natural dead space outwards and beyond the mouth and nose. An increase in the dead space volume during breathing increases carbon dioxide retention both at rest and under exertion and correspondingly the carbon dioxide partial pressure in the blood. This causes hypercapnia due to excess carbon dioxide build-up in the body.

This condition, also described as carbon dioxide retention, can cause effects such as breathlessness, headaches, dizziness and fatigue, as well as serious complications such as seizures or loss of consciousness. Hypoxia (decreased levels of oxygen in the blood) may result in additional non-physical effects such as confusion, disorientation, overall impaired cognitive abilities and decrease in psychomotor skills. This may also lead to hypoxemia (drop in oxygen below the normal limits).

A laboratory study published in 2013 by the "Annals of Occupational Hygiene" measured carbon dioxide (CO_2) levels in the breathing zones of thirty different models of N95 masks. The authors revealed that the average CO_2 concentrations ranged from 1.3% to 3.5%. These levels are in the vicinity of USA OSHA's (Occupational Safety and Health Administration) 15 minute limit for CO_2 (3%), 2.6-7.0 times OSHA's work shift limit for CO_2 (0.5% or 5000 ppm), 13-35 times the classroom limit for CO_2 in many countries (0.1% or 1000 ppm), about 30-80 times higher than the level of CO_2 in fresh air (0.04% or 400 ppm).

It is important to notice that healthcare workers wear masks for much longer than the short-term limit of 15 minutes. Very often they work 12 - 14 hour shifts with a N95 or N99 mask, the equivalent of the UK FFP2 and FFP3. Furthermore, all of the studies above were conducted in well-ventilated laboratories with CO_2 levels close to that of fresh air (400 ppm).

At this point I wish to discuss another example of diplodocus science: during my University studies the CO_2 levels of the classrooms were constantly monitored during the lectures. Reaching values of 1000 ppm constituted a major issue and the rooms had to be evacuated. At the same time the students were busy suffocating in their masks due to the re-inhaling of much higher and much more damaging levels of CO_2.

Inexplicably, this fact did not seem to raise any concern. We were also kept at freezing temperatures having to sit for hours with all the windows open in the midst of winter to allow ventilation and apparently decrease the chance of contracting COVID.

The result, in reality, was that several students that had managed to be perfectly healthy throughout the pandemic got sick with various respiratory diseases. Follow the science that is.

A lab study published in 2021 by the journal "Aerosol and Air Quality Research" measured CO_2 levels in the breathing zones of a surgical mask and a 3-layer cloth mask. The study found that the average CO_2 concentration in the cloth mask was 2,051 ppm - four times the 501 ppm level "when no mask was worn" and twice the 1,000 ppm classroom limit for CO_2 in many countries. The surgical mask provoked slightly higher results at 2,107 ppm, and this increased to 2,875 ppm when the subject walked on a treadmill at a moderate pace. The results of both studies observed levels of CO_2 comparable to the ones monitored in "sick building syndrome."

Another phenomenon that causes concern is the rebreathing of carbon dioxide due to the barrier created by the mask. A computer simulation published by the journal "Trauma and Emergency Care" in 2016 modelled a forty-seven year old female wearing an N95 mask and found that "60% of respired air re-entered the nasal cavity during the consecutive respiration cycle."

A study published by the journal "Anaesthesia" in 2006 measured CO_2 levels in the air exhaled by people wearing an N95 mask and found that CO_2 rose "due to rebreathing of air that is 'trapped' in the respirator, with the degree of rebreathing being proportional to the volume of the respirator ('dead space')." A computer simulation published by the journal "Physics of Fluids" in 2021 found that a N95 mask increases "CO_2 inhalation by approximately 7 times per breath compared with normal breathing" because the "mask restricts the ability of the exhaled air to mix with the ambient air, leading to an accumulation of CO_2 inside the mask."

Changes in blood gas parameters (O_2 and CO_2) are causes of clinically significant psychological and neurological effects. Masks also interfere with temperature regulation, impair the field of vision and are detrimental for verbal and non-verbal communication. As well as addressing the increased rebreathing of carbon dioxide due to the dead space, scientists also debate the influence of the increased breathing resistance when using masks.

In fact, science journals have proven that face masks restrict airflow. Experiments show an increase in airway resistance by a remarkable 126% on inhalation and 122% on exhalation with a N95 mask.

These are the first reported studies that demonstrate quantitatively and objectively the substantial impairment of nasal airflow in terms of increased breathing resistance with the use of N95 masks on human beings. Other studies have also shown that moisture in the N95 mask, due to regular inhalation and exhalation, increases the breathing resistance by a further 3% and can, consequently, increase the airway resistance up to two or three times the typical value.

This clearly shows the influence of masks on airway resistance. In this case, the mask acts as a disturbance factor in breathing and provokes compensatory reactions such as increase in breathing frequency and a feeling of breathlessness. This extra strain, due to the intensified breathing required to compensate the bigger resistance caused by the masks, also leads to increased exhaustion, a rise in heart rate, an augmented CO_2 production, significant respiratory impairment and a significant drop in oxygen saturation in about 75% of all study results.

Consequently, a substantial portion of people who wear masks report difficulty in breathing.

In another study from 2011, all tested masks caused a significantly measurable increase in discomfort and a feeling of exhaustion in the twenty seven subjects during prolonged usage.

These symptoms lead to additional stress for the workers and, consequently, further possibility of distraction and errors.

A study conducted in fourteen Vietnamese hospitals and published in 2015 by the journal "BMJ Open" found that 18.3% of healthcare workers who wore a cloth or surgical mask "reported breathing problems."

A study published in 2019 by the journal "BMC Infectious Diseases" found that 12% of hospital workers who wore a surgical mask for one shift reported "breathing difficulty."

A study published in 2021 by the "International Journal of Bioinformatics and Biomedical Engineering" found that 22% of 183 medical students at a college in India "experienced breathing difficulty while wearing N95, surgical, or cloth masks".

Increase in respiratory rate, increase in heart rate, decrease in oxygen saturation, and increase in carbon dioxide partial pressure cause fatigue, headaches, dizziness and impaired thinking as well as a sensation of heat and itching due to moisture of the masks and additionally intensification of subjective chest complaints.

The mask-induced adverse reactions are relatively minor at first glance, but repeated exposure over longer periods of time to those pathogenetic processes is relevant. The statistically significant results found in the studies with tangible differences between mask wearers and people without masks are clinically meaningful. They give an indication that with repeated and prolonged exposure to harmful physical, chemical, biological, physiological and psychological conditions individuals can develop diseases such as high blood pressure and arteriosclerosis, coronary heart disease and neurological diseases.

Even small increases in carbon dioxide can create headaches, irritation of the respiratory tract, asthma, vascular damage and neuropathological and cardiovascular consequences. Slightly but persistently increased heart rates encourage oxidative stress with endothelial dysfunction, high blood pressure, cardiac dysfunction and damage to blood vessels supplying the brain.

In 2012, an experiment showed that walking whilst wearing a mask significantly increased heart rates (average 9.4 beats per minute) and breathing rates. These physiological changes were accompanied by increased carbon dioxide levels as well as respiratory difficulties in the mask wearers compared to the control group.

In a recent experimental comparative study from 2020, twelve healthy volunteers under surgical masks as well as under N95 masks experienced measurable impairments in the measured lung function parameters as well as cardiopulmonary capacity during moderate to heavy physical exertion compared to exertion without masks. The mask-induced amplified airway resistance led to increased respiratory work with augmented oxygen consumption and demand, both on the respiratory muscles and the heart. Breathing was significantly impeded and participants reported mild pain. The scientists concluded that the cardiac compensation due to the defective pulmonary functioning which is still tolerable in healthy people, is probably no longer possible in patients with reduced cardiac output. This also gives an indication of the effect of masks on sick and elderly people even without exertion.

In COPD patients, after only 10 minutes of mask-wearing, a significant increase in heart rate, increase in systolic blood pressure and carbon dioxide, even at rest, was noticed. This was also accompanied by a decrease in oxygen saturation.

Furthermore, face coverings can inflate the risk of acquiring pneumonia and other respiratory diseases.

One study found for example that as little as four hours of wearing a cloth or plastic mask increased vulnerability to bacterial infection. There are also the largely unknown risks from the inhalation of micro-plastics and the exposure to contaminants in the textiles which will be explored in later chapters.

Cardio-Pulmonary Stress

An array of science journals have published studies showing that exercising with a mask causes heart and lung stress, negatively impacts performance, and may have caused some deaths.

A study published in 2020 by the journal "Clinical Research in Cardiology" measured effects of surgical and N95 masks on twelve healthy males aged thirty-two to forty-two as they exercised vigorously.

The "sample primarily consisted of physicians working at a university hospital who are very familiar with medical masks and have a positive attitude towards personal protection." The study found that: "ventilation, cardiopulmonary exercise capacity and comfort are reduced by surgical masks and highly impaired by N95 masks"; the masks "have a marked negative impact on cardiopulmonary capacity that significantly impairs strenuous physical and occupational activities"; the masks also have "a significant impact on pulmonary parameters" when resting; the masks "significantly impair the quality of life of their wearer" by causing "breathing resistance, heat, tightness," and "severe subjective discomfort during exercise."

A study published in 2020 by the "Asia-Pacific Journal of Sports Medicine, Arthroscopy, Rehabilitation and Technology" measured effects of wearing a surgical mask while exercising moderately. The sample consisted of twenty three people aged twenty one to sixty who walked on a treadmill for six minutes to simulate "outdoor recreational hiking on an uphill slope at a comfortable pace." The study found that the mask: "significantly increased their heart rates by an average of 4.4 beats per minute"; "significantly increased" their rates of perceived exertion"; caused "higher physiological responses possibly due to restricted ventilation, heavier breathing, and sympathetic responses"; caused "an uncomfortable feeling of dyspnoea (shortness of breath)" for some volunteers; increased "the physiological burden on their bodies, especially in those with multiple underlying comorbidities."

A 2020 paper in the journal "Medical Hypotheses" found: "Recently, there have been case reports of Sudden Cardiac Death (SCD) occurring during exercise with face masks."

Exercise "with face masks may increase the risk of SCD via several mechanisms" detailed in the paper. They advised "avoidance of a face mask during high intensity exercise, or if wearing of a mask is mandatory, exercise intensity should remain low to avoid precipitation of lethal arrhythmias (heartbeat irregularities)."

They could not "exclude the possibility of a fatal cardiac event caused by a mask during low intensity exercise especially for people with heart disease".

A study published in 2021 by the journal "Applied Sciences" measured effects of a surgical mask on seventy-two recreational athletes as they ran at their maximum speed for 50 meters and 400 meters. The study found that the mask: "increased blood lactate concentration, sympathetic autonomic modulation, perceived exertion, perceived stress, and decreased blood oxygen saturation and negatively affected their running performance by increasing the average time to complete a 50 metres race by 12.51% and a 400 metres race by 19.09%".

A study published in 2021 by the "British Journal of Sports Medicine" measured effects of a cloth mask on thirty healthy adults aged eighteen to twenty nine years as they ran at max speed on a treadmill. The study found that the mask: "led to a 14% reduction in exercise time"; "reduced their "maximal oxygen consumption by 29%"; caused the participants to feel "increasingly short of breath and claustrophobic at higher exercise intensities."

Most of the diplodocus science ignores all of the above studies and normally cites the ones that use only low exercise intensities, short exposure times, imprecise measurements or exclude people with "cardiac or respiratory conditions" or deems as acceptable oxygen saturations levels below 92% when the normal value should not fall under 96%. Another way of deceiving can be seen in the following interpretation of a study. Published in 2021 by the "Annals of the American Thoracic Society", it measured the effects of a surgical mask on fifteen healthy doctors (average age of thirty-one) and fifteen patients (average age of seventy-two) with severe chronic obstructive pulmonary disease (COPD) as they rested and after they walked. Regarding the results of the study and the presentation of them: the study found "no major changes" of "clinical significance" in the oxygen saturation of the participants' blood or the CO_2 concentration of their exhaled breath when they wore a mask for thirty minutes while resting.

Concerning this timeframe, a 2018 paper in the journal "Nature" documents that the physiological impacts of elevated CO_2 on office workers and pilots do not manifest until after 40 to 60 minutes. The walking test for this study was conducted over six minutes and only on the COPD patients while they wore masks. The study did not establish a baseline for walking "without a mask" because "our institution required everyone to wear masks in the room where the walking test was performed".

The study found that the COPD patients "did not exhibit major physiologic changes" from walking with a mask "as a group." Two of the patients, however, required "supplemental oxygen" during or after the walk, and the authors buried in a table the fact that one of the patients experienced a 19.0% drop in their oxygen saturation.

According to the Centre for Evidence-Based Medicine at Oxford University, "even a small decline in oxygen saturation during exercise should alert the clinician and a drop of 3% should be cause for serious concern, regardless of the amount of exercise needed to produce it."

The authors closed their paper by claiming, "It is important to inform the public that the discomfort associated with mask use should not lead to unsubstantiated safety concerns as this may attenuate the application of a practice proved to improve public health."

In short, the authority's risk-free portrayal of exercising while masked is false and dangerous.

Furthermore, people who have acted in accord with the facts of this matter have paid a heavy price. Many sport coaches lost their jobs for refusing to make their athletes wear masks.

Heat & Discomfort

The heat, humidity, and other discomforts of wearing a mask are not merely annoyances. This is because "heat and moisture trapping beneath surgical face masks," as explained in the "Journal of Hospital Infection", may cause "decreased mental and physical performance."

Measured by the heat index, the interiors of masks can be overheating, even in climate-controlled rooms. A study published in 2012 by the journal "Respiratory Physiology & Neurobiology" found that when "young, healthy adults" engaged in "low-moderate" intensity exercise with a surgical mask, the air inside the masks averaged 32.74°C at 91% relative humidity. This equates to a heat index of 52.9°C. For comparison, the air in the room where the test was conducted was 21.47°C at 23% relative humidity, a heat index of 20.55°C.

Neurological Side Effects and Dangers

A series of experiments published by the "Journal of Experimental Psychology" in 2008 found that "an entirely irrelevant distraction factor can interfere with task performance" by causing "increased error rates" and "response times."

For people working in hospitals, factories, and offices where mental sharpness or attention to detail are vital to safety or performance, the discomforts and distractions of masks could make the difference between life and death. This is not mere hypothetical because the fatal line can be easily crossed in certain environments.

Based on a systematic literature review published by the "Journal of Patient Safety" in 2013, "there are at least 210,000 lethal" errors in US hospitals each year, and "the true number" is "estimated at more than 400,000 per year."

CO_2 concentrations in surgical and cloth masks may impair certain high-level brain functions.

A study of 22 people published in 2012 by the journal "Environmental Health Perspectives" found the following impacts from 2.5 hours of CO_2 exposure at 2,500 ppm: "Large and statistically significant reductions" in seven out of nine categories of decision-making performance in a test of "real-world day-to-day challenges." These included measures of initiative, information usage, strategic thinking, and other factors associated with life success; losses in five categories of decision-making performance that sunk "to levels associated with marginal or dysfunctional performance."; a gain in one category of decision-making performance (focus), which is common among people who have "mild-to-moderate head injuries" or are "under the influence of alcohol."

This is because such events cause people "to become highly focused on smaller details at the expense of the big picture."

A study of 30 active commercial aircraft pilots published in 2018 by the journal "Nature" found the following impacts from CO_2 exposure in a flight simulator at levels ranging from 700 to 2,500 ppm:

Pilot examiners determined that the pilots' odds of properly executing complex flight manoeuvres significantly decreased at a CO_2 level of 2,500 ppm.

"Passing rates were twice as high at 700 ppm and 1500 ppm during a take-off with an engine fire than at 2500 ppm, and four times higher at 700 ppm during a rejected take-off than at 2500 ppm."

"The effect of CO_2 on passing rates became more pronounced the longer the pilots were in the simulator, with the response between CO_2 exposure and passing rate becoming apparent after 40 minutes." This response effect, as explained by epidemiologist Sydney Pettygrove, "is one in which increasing levels of exposure are associated with either an increasing or a decreasing risk of the outcome." When this pattern occurs, it "is considered strong evidence for a causal relationship between the exposure and the outcome."

Some examples of the pilots' failures at 2,500 ppm included: "Did not deploy the reversers/did not call"; "No callout/ disconnected auto-brakes" and "did not set parking brake."

In other fields, in a scientific evaluation of syncope (loss of consciousness caused by decrease of blood flow to the brain) in an operating theatre, 36 of 77 affected persons (47%) were associated with wearing a mask even though other factors could not be ruled out as contributory causes.

In their level three evidence review, neurologists from Israel, the UK and the USA state that a mask is unsuitable for epileptics because it can trigger hyperventilation. Furthermore, the use of a mask significantly increases the respiratory rate by about 15 to 20%. An increase in breathing frequency leading to hyperventilation is known to be used for provocation in the diagnosis of epilepsy and causes seizure-equivalent EEG (electroencephalogram) changes in 80% of patients with generalised epilepsy and in up to 28% of focal epileptics.

Physicians from New York studied the effects of wearing surgical N95 masks among medical personnel in a sample of 343 participants surveyed using standardised, anonymised questionnaires. Wearing the masks caused detectable physical adverse effects such as impaired cognition (24% of wearers) and headaches in 71.4% of the participants. Of these, 28% persisted and required medication. Headache occurred in 15.2% under one hour of wearing, in 30.6% after one hour of wearing and in 29.7% after three hours of wearing. Thus, the effect intensified with increasing wearing time.

As a result of mask use confusion, disorientation and drowsiness, reduced motor abilities and reduced reactivity and overall impaired performance have also been documented in other studies.

The scientists explain these neurological impairments with a mask-induced latent drop in blood gas oxygen levels (hypoxia) or a latent increase in blood gas carbon dioxide levels (hypercapnia). In view of the scientific data, this connection also appears to be indisputable.

In a mask experiment from 2020, significant impaired thinking and impaired concentration were found for all mask types used (fabric, surgical and N95 masks) after only 100 minutes of wearing the mask. The thought disorders correlated significantly with a drop in oxygen saturation during mask use.

Gynaecological Side Effects and Dangers

For a pregnant woman and her unborn child, there is a metabolic need for a foetal-maternal carbon dioxide (CO_2) gradient. The mother's blood carbon dioxide level should always be lower than that of the unborn child in order to ensure the diffusion of CO_2 from the foetal blood into the maternal circulation via the placenta.

Therefore, mask-related phenomena described above, such as the measurable changes in respiratory physiology with increased breathing resistance, increased dead space volume and the retention of exhaled carbon dioxide (CO_2) are fundamental factors. If CO_2 is increasingly rebreathed under masks, this manifestation could, even with subliminal carbon dioxide increases, act as a disturbing variable of the foetal–maternal CO_2 gradient increasing over time of exposure and, therefore, develop clinical relevance, also with regard to a reduced compensation reserve of the expectant mothers.

In a comparative study, twenty two pregnant women wearing N95 masks during 20 minutes of exercise showed significantly higher percutaneous CO_2 values, with average $PtcCO_2$ values of 33.3 mmHg compared to 31.3 mmHg in another twenty two pregnant women without masks. The heat sensation of the expectant mothers was also significantly increased with masks.

Accordingly, in another intervention study, researchers demonstrated that breathing through an N95 mask (FFP2 equivalent) impeded gas exchange in 20 pregnant women at rest and during exercise, causing additional stress on their metabolic system. Under a N95 mask, twenty pregnant women showed a decrease in oxygen uptake capacity (VO_2) of about 14% and a decrease in carbon dioxide output capacity (VCO_2) of about 18% which is statistically significant.

Corresponding meaningful changes in exhaled oxygen and carbon dioxide equivalents were also documented with increases in exhaled carbon dioxide ($FeCO_2$) and decreases in exhaled oxygen (FeO_2), which were explained by an altered metabolism due to respiratory mask obstruction.

In experiments with predominantly short mask application times, neither the mothers nor the foetuses showed statistically significant increases in heart rates or changes in respiratory rates and oxygen saturation values. However, the exact effects of prolonged mask use in pregnant women remain unclear overall. Therefore, in pregnant women, extended use of surgical and N95 masks is viewed critically.

In addition, it is unclear whether the substances contained in industrially manufactured masks that can be inhaled over longer periods of time (e.g. formaldehyde as an ingredient of the textile and thiram as an ingredient of the ear bands) are teratogenic (something that can cause or raise the risk for a birth defect in a baby).

Dermatological Side Effects and Dangers

Masks cover the mouth and nose and inevitably, this leads not only to a measurable temperature rise, but also to a severe increase in humidity due to condensation of the exhaled air, which in turn changes considerably the natural skin environment of perioral and paranasal areas. It also measurably increases redness, pH-values and fluid loss through the epithelium decreased hydration and sebum production. Pre-existing skin diseases are not only perpetuated by these changes, but also exacerbated. In general, the skin becomes more susceptible to infections and acne.

This picture shows what happens to my youngest daughter when she wears a face mask for only few hours.

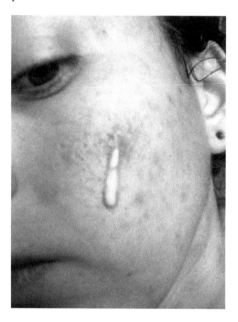

This phenomenon is confirmed by the authors of an experimental study that were able to prove a disturbed barrier function of the skin after only four hours of wearing a mask in 20 healthy volunteers, both for surgical masks and for N95 masks.

In addition, germs (bacteria, fungi and viruses) accumulate on the outside and inside of the masks due to the warm and moist environment. This can cause clinically relevant fungal, bacterial or viral infections. The unusual increase in the detection of rhinoviruses in the sentinel studies of the German Robert Koch Institute (RKI) from 2020 could be another indication of this phenomenon.

Furthermore, a region of the skin that is not evolutionarily adapted to such stimuli is subjected to increased mechanical stress. The above mentioned events cause dermatological effects and mask related adverse skin reactions and irritations like acne, rashes and itching.

A Chinese research group reported skin irritation and itching when using N95 masks among 542 test participants and also a correlation between skin damage and time of exposure (68.9% at ≤6 hours/day and 81.7% at >6 hours/day).

A New York study evaluated in a random sample of 343 participants the effects of frequent N95 mask wearing among healthcare workers during the COVID-19 pandemic. Wearing the masks caused headache in 71.4% of participants, in addition to drowsiness in 23.6%, detectable skin damage in 51% and acne in 53% of mask users.

On the one hand, direct mechanical skin lesions occur on the nose and cheekbones due to sheer force, especially when masks are frequently put on and taken off.

Masks also create an unnaturally moist and warm local skin environment. In fact, in another study in which test individuals wore masks for one hour scientists were able to demonstrate a significant increase in humidity and temperature in the covered facial area. The relative humidity under the masks was measured with a sensor. The sensation of humidity and temperature in the facial area is more crucial for well-being than other body regions as will be explained in detail in chapter 7. This can increase discomfort under the masks. In addition, the increase in temperature favours bacterial growth.

The pressure of the masks also causes an obstruction of the physiological flow of lymph and blood vessels in the face, with the consequence of increased disturbance of skin function and ultimately also contributing to acne in up to 53% of all wearers and other skin irritations in up to 51% of all wearers.

Other researchers examined 322 participants with N95 masks in an observational study and detected acne in up to 59.6% of them, itching in 51.4% and redness in 35.8% as side effects.

In up to 19.6% (273) of the 1393 wearers of different masks (community masks, surgical, N95 masks), itching could be objectified in one study, in 9% of the cases even severely. An atopic predisposition (allergy tendency) correlated with the risk of itching as well as the length of use.

In another dermatological study from 2020, 96.9% of 876 users of all mask types (community masks, surgical masks, N95 masks) confirmed adverse problems with a significant increase in itching (7.7%), accompanied by fogging-up of glasses (21.3%), flushing (21.3%), slurred speech (12.3%) and difficulty breathing.

Apart from an increased incidence of acne due to masks, contact eczema and urticaria are generally detected in connection with hypersensitivities to ingredients of the industrially manufactured masks (surgical mask and N95) such as formaldehyde (ingredient of the textile) and thiram (ingredient of the ear bands). The hazardous substance thiram, originally a pesticide and corrosive, is used in the rubber industry as an optimisation accelerator. Formaldehyde is a biocide and carcinogen and is used as a disinfectant in the industry.

Isolated permanent hyperpigmentation as a result of post-inflammatory or pigmented contact dermatitis has also been described by dermatologists after prolonged mask use.

ENT (ear, nose, throat) and dental side effects and dangers

Dentist are reporting about the negative effects of masks and are calling the phenomena "mask mouth", a disease that could have serious consequences, including death.

"Gum disease, or periodontal disease, will eventually lead to strokes and an increased risk of heart attacks," warns Marc Sclafani, a dentist and co-founder of One Manhattan Dental.

"We're seeing inflammation in people's gums that have been healthy forever, and cavities in people who have never had them before," adds Rob Ramondi, another dentist and co-founder at One Manhattan Dental.

According to Ramondi, roughly half of his patients are suffering from health problems due to wearing a mask and the complications can be extremely severe.

"About 50 percent of our patients are being impacted by this.'"

Wearing a face covering breeds bacteria in front of the mouth and nose, where pathogens flourish in a warm, moist environment. These pathogens then enter the mouth and body, creating disease.

The symptoms are gingivitis (inflammation of the gums), halitosis (bad breath), candidiasis (fungal infestation of the mucous membranes with Candida albicans) and cheilitis (inflammation of the lips), especially of the corners of the mouth. Those are attributed to the excessive and improper use of masks. The main trigger of the mentioned oral diseases is an increased dry mouth due to a reduced saliva flow (and saliva is what fights the bacteria and cleanse the teeth)- and increased breathing through the open mouth under the mask.

Dry mouth is scientifically proven to occur as a consequence of mask wearing. The bad habit of breathing through the mouth while wearing a mask is a natural outcome that arises in order to compensate for the increased breathing resistance, especially when inhaling, lack of oxygen and excess recycled carbon dioxide waste inside the mask. In turn, the outer skin moisture with altered skin flora, instigates the inflammation of the lips and corners of the mouth (cheilitis). The physiological internal moisture with external dryness in the oral cavity converts into internal dryness with external moisture.

Coronavirus masks are killing people, dentists warn, in the coming months and years, expect to see a pandemic of oral health problems, heart problems, and early death caused by mask mouth. The establishment will blame it all on COVID, of course, but do not be fooled: masks are the culprit.

"Patients are coming into us like, 'Wow, my breath smells, I need a cleaning.' But when you smell the bad breath, you either already have periodontal disease or you have a lot of bacteria that's sitting on your tongue because of dry mouth" Sclafani further explains.

Furthermore, ENT physicians recently discovered a new form of irritant rhinitis due to N95 mask use in forty - six patients. They performed endoscopies and nasal irrigations on mask wearers, which were subsequently assessed pathologically. They found statistically significant evidence of mask-induced rhinitis and itching and swelling of the mucous membranes as well as increased sneezing. Endoscopies showed an increased secretion and evidence of inhaled mask polypropylene fibres as the trigger of mucosal irritation.

In a study of 221 health care workers, ENT physicians diagnosed a voice disorder in 33% of mask users. The parameter that measures voice disorders, was on average 5.72 higher in these mask users.

The mask not only acted as an acoustic filter, provoking excessively loud speech, it also seemed to trigger impaired vocal cord coordination because the mask compromises the pressure gradients required for undisturbed speech. The researchers concluded from their findings that masks could pose a potential risk of triggering new voice disorders as well as exacerbating existing ones.

Microbiological Consequences and Foreign/Self-Contamination

Masks cause retention of moisture. Poor filtration performance and incorrect use of surgical and community masks, as well as their frequent reuse, imply an increased risk of infection.

The warm and humid microclimate environment created by and in masks without the presence of protective mechanisms such as antibodies, paves the way for an ideal growth and breeding ground for various pathogens such as bacteria, fungi and viruses to accumulate underneath the masks. The measurable germ density is proportional to the length of mask wearing. After only two hours, the pathogen density increases almost tenfold in experimental observation studies.

From a microbiological and epidemiological point of view, in everyday use, masks pose a high risk of contamination. This can occur as foreign contamination but also as self-contamination.

On the one hand, germs are sucked in or attach themselves to the masks through convection currents. On the other hand, potential infectious agents from the nasopharynx accumulate excessively on both the outside and inside of the mask during breathing. This is compounded by contact with contaminated hands.

Since masks are constantly penetrated by germ-containing breath and the pathogen reproduction rate is higher outside mucous membranes, potential infectious pathogens accumulate excessively on the outside and inside of masks. On and in the masks, there are quite serious, potentially disease-causing bacteria and fungi such as E. coli (54% of all germs detected), Staphylococcus aureus (25%), Candida (6%), Klebsiella (5%), Enterococci (4%), Pseudomonads (3%), Enterobacter (2%) and Micrococcus (1%) even detectable in large quantities.

In another microbiological study, the bacterium Staphylococcus aureus (57%) and the fungus Aspergillus (31% of all fungi detected) were found to be the dominant germs in 230 surgical masks examined.

After more than six hours of use, the following viruses were found in descending order on 148 masks worn by medical personnel: adenovirus, bocavirus, respiratory syncytial virus and influenza viruses.

It is also problematic that moisture distributes these potential pathogens in the form of tiny droplets via capillary action on and in the mask, whereby further proliferation in the sense of self and foreign contamination by the aerosols can then occur internally and externally with every breath. In this regard, it is also known from the literature that masks are responsible for a disproportionate production of fine particles in the environment and, surprisingly, much more so than in people without masks.

It was shown that all mask-wearing subjects released significantly more smaller particles of size 0.3–0.5 μm into the air than mask-less people, both when breathing, speaking and coughing (fabric, surgical, N95 masks). The increase in the detection of rhinoviruses in the sentinel studies of the German RKI from 2020 could be a further indication of this phenomenon, as masks were consistently used by the general population in public spaces in that year.

In 2021, the "Journal of Transport & Health" published a covert study of 182 passengers on subways and local trains in the area of Paris, France. It found that during a median observation time of 8 minutes, 48% of people touched their masks, and they did so at an average rate of 15 times per hour. The study also revealed an "Increased tendency to touch the face while wearing a face mask" and noted that this "might increase the risk of transmission and self-contamination."

The implications of mask touching are much broader than transmission and contamination. This is because momentary distractions (like adjusting a mask) can hamper job performance.

Epidemiological Consequences

A major risk of mask use in the general public is the creation of a false sense of security with regard to protection against viral infections, especially in the sense of a falsely assumed strong self-protection.

Disregarding infection risks may not only neglect aspects of source control, but also result in other disadvantages. Although there are quite a few professional positive accounts of the widespread use of masks in the general populace, most of the serious and evident scientific reports conclude that the general obligation to wear masks conveys a false sense of security. This leads to neglect of those measures that, according to the WHO, have a higher level of effectiveness than mask-wearing: social distancing and hand hygiene. Researchers were able to provide statistically significant evidence of a false sense of security and more risky behaviour when wearing masks in an experimental setting.

Decision makers in many countries informed their citizens in March 2020 or early in the pandemic that people without symptoms should not use a medical mask, as this created a false sense of security. The recommendation was ultimately changed in many countries. Many governments pointed out that wearers of community masks cannot rely on them to protect them or others from transmission of SARS-CoV-2.

However, scientists not only complain about the lack of evidence for fabric masks in the scope of a pandemic, but also about the high permeability of fabric masks with particles and the potential risk of infection they pose. Ordinary fabric masks with a 97% penetration for particle dimensions of

≥0.3 µm are in stark contrast to medical-type surgical masks with a 44% penetration. In contrast, the N95 mask has a penetration rate of less than 0.01% for particles ≥ 0.3 µm in the laboratory experiment.

For the clinical setting in hospitals and outpatient clinics, the WHO guidelines recommend only surgical masks for influenza viruses for the entire patient treatment except for the strongly aerosol-generating measures, for which finer filtering masks of the type N95 are suggested. However, the WHO's endorsement of specific mask types is not evidence-based due to the lack of high-quality studies in the health sector. More on this in chapter six.

In a laboratory experiment, it was demonstrated that both surgical masks and N95 masks have deficits in protection against SARS-CoV-2 and influenza viruses using virus-free aerosols. In this study, the FFP2-equivalent N95 mask performed significantly better in protection (8–12 times more effective) than the surgical mask, but neither mask type established reliable, hypothesis-generated protection against corona and influenza viruses. Both mask types could be penetrated unhindered by aerosol particles with a diameter of 0.08 to 0.2 µm. Both the SARS-CoV-2 pathogens with a size of 0.06 to 0.14 µm and the influenza viruses with 0.08 to 0.12 µm are unfortunately well below the mask pore sizes.

The filtering capacity of the N95 mask up to 0.3 µm is usually not achieved by surgical masks and community masks. However, aerosol droplets, which have a diameter of 0.09 to 3 µm in size, are supposed to serve as a transport medium for viruses. These also penetrate the medical masks by 40%. Often, there is also a poor fit between the face and the mask, which further impairs their function and safety. The accumulation of aerosol droplets on the mask is problematic. Not only they absorb nanoparticles such as viruses, but they also follow the airflow when inhaling and exhaling, causing them to be carried further in the deepest areas of the lungs.

In addition, a physical decay process has been described for aerosol droplets at increasing temperatures, which also occurs under a mask. This process can lead to a decrease in size of the fine water droplets up to the diameter of a virus. The masks filter larger aerosol droplets but cannot do the same with smaller, potentially virus-containing aerosol droplets of less than 0.2 µm and hence cannot stop the spread of COVID.

Similarly, in an in vivo comparative study of N95 and surgical masks, there were no significant differences in influenza virus infection rates.

A Swiss textile lab test of various masks available on the market to the general public recently confirmed that most mask types filter aerosols insufficiently. For all but one of the eight reusable fabric mask types tested, the filtration efficacy according to EN149 was always less than 70% for particles of 1 µm in size. For disposable masks, only half of all eight mask types tested were efficient enough at filtering to retain 70% of particles 1 µm in size.

A recent experimental study even demonstrated that all mask-wearing people (surgical, N95, fabric masks) release significantly and proportionately smaller particles of size 0.3 to 0.5 µm into the air than mask-less people, both when breathing, speaking and coughing. According to this, the masks act like nebulisers and contribute to the production of very fine aerosols. Smaller particles, however, spread faster and further than large ones for physical reasons. Of particular interest in this experimental reference study was the finding that a test subject wearing a single-layer fabric mask was also able to release a total of 384% more particles (of various sizes) when breathing than a person without.

It is not only the aforementioned functional weaknesses of the masks themselves that lead to problems, but also their use. This increases the risk of a false sense of security.

According to the literature, mistakes are made by both healthcare workers and lay people when using masks as hygienically correct mask use is by no means intuitive. Overall, 65% of healthcare professionals and as many as 78% of the general population, use masks incorrectly. With both surgical masks and N95 masks, adherence to the rules of use is impaired and not adequately followed due to reduced wearability with heat discomfort and skin irritation.

This is exacerbated by the accumulation of carbon dioxide due to the dead space (especially under the N95 masks) with the resulting headaches described. Increased heart rate, itching and feelings of dampness also lead to reduced safety and quality during use (see also social and occupational health side effects and hazards). For this reason, masks are even considered as a general risk for infection in the general population, which does not come close to imitating the strict hygiene rules of hospitals and doctors' surgeries: the supposed safety, thus, becomes a safety risk itself.

In a meta-analysis commissioned by the WHO, no effect of masks in the context of influenza virus pandemic prevention could be demonstrated. In 14 randomised controlled trials, no reduction in the transmission of laboratory-confirmed influenza infections was shown. Due to the similar size and distribution pathways of the virus species (influenza and generic coronavirus), the data can also be transferred to SARS-CoV-2. Nevertheless, a combination of occasional mask-wearing with adequate handwashing caused a slight reduction in infections for influenza in one study. However, since no separation of hand hygiene and masks was achieved in this study, the protective effect can rather be attributed to hand hygiene in view of the aforementioned data.

A recently published large prospective Danish study comparing mask wearers and non-mask wearers in terms of their infection rates with SARS-CoV-2 could not demonstrate any statistically significant differences between the groups.

Paediatric Side Effects and Hazards

Children are a particularly vulnerable category and may be more likely to receive inappropriate treatment or additional harm due to mask wearing. It can be assumed that the potential adverse mask effects described for adults are all the more valid for children.

Special attention must be paid to the respiration of children, which represents a critical and vulnerable physiological variable due to higher oxygen demand, increased hypoxia susceptibility of the central nervous system, lower respiratory reserve, smaller airways with a stronger increase in resistance when the flow of air is narrowed. Mask wearing can cause anything between respiratory arrest to bradycardia in the event of oxygen deficiency.

The masks currently used for children are exclusively adult masks manufactured in smaller geometric dimensions and had neither been specially tested nor approved for this purpose.

In an experimental British research study, the masks frequently led to feelings of heat and breathing problems in 100 school children between 8 and 11 years of age especially during physical exertion, which is why the protective equipment was taken off by 24% of the children during physical activity. The exclusion criteria for this mask experiment were lung disease, cardiovascular impairment and claustrophobia.

Scientists from Singapore were able to demonstrate in their study published in the journal "Nature" that 106 children aged between 7 and 14 years who wore FFP2 masks for only 5 minutes showed an increase in the inspiratory and expiratory CO_2 levels, indicating disturbed respiratory physiology.

However, a disturbed respiratory physiology in children can have long-term disease-relevant consequences. Slightly elevated CO_2 levels are known to increase heart rate, blood pressure, headache, fatigue and concentration disorders.

Accordingly, the following conditions were listed as exclusion criteria for mask use: any cardiopulmonary disease including but not limited to: asthma, bronchitis, cystic fibrosis, congenital heart disease, emphysema; any condition that may be aggravated by physical exertion, including but not limited to: exercise-induced asthma; lower respiratory tract infections (pneumonia, bronchitis within the last 2 weeks), anxiety disorders, diabetes, hypertension or epilepsy/attack disorder; any physical disability due to medical, orthopaedic or neuromuscular disease; any acute upper respiratory illness or symptomatic rhinitis (nasal obstruction, runny nose or sneezing); any condition with deformity that affects the fit of the mask (e.g. increased facial hair, craniofacial deformities, etc.).

It is also important to emphasise the possible effects of masks in neurological diseases, as described earlier in the case of adults.

Both masks and face shields caused fear in 46% of children (37 out of 80) in a scientific study. If children are given the choice of whether the doctor examining them should wear a mask they reject this in 49% of the cases. Along with their parents, the children prefer the practitioner to wear a face visor.

A recent observational study of tens of thousands of mask-wearing children in Germany objectify complaints of headaches (53%), difficulty concentrating (50%), joylessness (49%), learning difficulties (38%) and fatigue (37%) of the 25,930 children evaluated. Of the children observed, 25% had new onset anxiety and even nightmares. In children, the threat scenarios generated by the environment are further maintained via masks, in some cases, even further increased and in this way, existing stress is intensified through the insurgence and prolongation of subconscious fears.

This can in turn lead to an increase in psychosomatic and stress-related illnesses. For example, according to an evaluation, 60% of mask wearers showed stress levels of the highest grade 10 on a scale of 1 to a maximum of 10. Less than 10% of the mask wearers surveyed had a stress level lower than 8 out of a possible 10.

As children are considered a special group, the WHO also issued a separate guideline on the use of masks in children in the community in August 2020, explicitly advising policy makers and national authorities, given the limited evidence, that the benefits of mask use in children must be weighed up against the potential harms associated with mask use. This includes feasibility and discomfort, as well as social and communication concerns.

According to experts, masks block the foundation of human communication and the exchange of emotions and not only hinder learning but deprive children of the positive effects of smiling, laughing and emotional mimicry. The effectiveness of masks in children as a viral protection is controversial, and there is a lack of evidence for their widespread use in children; this is also addressed in more detail by the scientists of the German University of Bremen in some of their student's thesis and in chapter nine.

Most of world institutions and governments disregarded any of those recommendations and coerced children to wear masks in schools and public venues through blanket mandates causing enormous harm which is, as yet, impossible to quantify or forecast.

Increased risk of falls in the elderly

By blocking parts of the lower peripheral visual field, and causing spectacles to steam up, masks will increase the risk of falls in older people with ongoing mobility difficulties. Injuries, such as fractured femurs, are more prevalent in the elderly. Requiring face coverings from this demographic, the most regular visitors to healthcare facilities, can only exacerbate the risk.

The October 2020 study by the BMJ states the following:

"Although guidance recommends that older adults wear masks because they are an at-risk group, it is this population for whom the effects of masks on walking safety are likely to be most pronounced. Aside from obstructing vision for glasses wearers (by causing spectacles to fog up), face masks invariably block parts of the lower peripheral visual field, even in people who do not wear glasses. Visual information from the lower peripheral field is important for detecting and avoiding nearby hazards, and for placing our steps safely. Wearing a face mask reduces the wearer's opportunity to use this important sensory information during walking and may therefore increase the chance of tripping or falling. Evidence exists that multifocal glasses (which similarly obstruct lower visual field, through blurring) can reduce safety when negotiating obstacles and stairs.

It might seem logical to advise people to look down at their feet more often while wearing a face mask. This would provide the visual information that they would normally obtain through lower peripheral vision when looking ahead. Indeed, such advice is beginning to emerge. While intuitive, we argue that this advice is flawed. To understand why, it is important to consider the two functions for which vision is used when walking. Firstly, vision is used to detect obstacles and plan a safe walking route, especially in older adults. Looking down more often makes it more difficult to plan ahead. Recent research using eye tracking technology shows that older adults make greater stepping errors when looking down towards their feet compared with when looking ahead and visually previewing potential trip hazards.

Secondly, maintaining balance requires visual information (particularly from the periphery) to be integrated with other sensory inputs. This is facilitated by minimising head and eye movements during walking, to provide a stable visual "anchor" that serves as the predominant source of sensory information for regulating balance. Using vision in this manner is particularly important for older adults. Looking down more often is in direct conflict with this strategy. It could even cause serious instability as it requires frequent and large amplitude movements of the head and eyes, which could lead to a mismatch between visual and vestibular feedback.

In short, a recommendation to simply "look down" when wearing a mask may paradoxically impair stability by disrupting the finely tuned system through which vision is used to maintain walking safety. This will affect not only older adults, but anyone for whom balance is particularly reliant on vision, such as people with Parkinson's disease or diabetic sensory neuropathy.

At risk groups should be advised to "take their time" rather than "look down." Specifically, people should take their time before starting to walk and then walk more slowly. This will ensure that they have enough time to detect upcoming trip hazards and plan a safe route."

Sports Medicine: Side Effects and Dangers

According to the literature, masks have no performance-enhancing effects.

In an experimental reference study, a training mask that supposedly mimics altitude conditions had only training effects on the respiratory muscles. However, mask wearers showed significantly lower oxygen saturation values during exercise (SpO_2 of 94% for mask wearers versus 96% for mask-less), which can be explained by an increased dead space volume and resistance during breathing. The measured oxygen saturation values were significantly lower than the normal values in the group of mask wearers, which is clinically relevant.

The proven adaptation effect of the respiratory muscles in healthy athletes clearly suggests that masks have a disruptive effect on respiratory physiology.

In another intervention study on mask use in weightlifters, researchers documented statistically significant effects of reduced attention and a slowed maximum speed of movement detectable by means of sensors. The researchers concluded that mask use in sport is not without risks. As a secondary finding, they also detected a significant decrease in oxygen saturation SpO_2 when performing special weight-lifting exercises in the mask group after only one minute of exercise compared to the mask-free group. The proven tendency of the masks to shift oxygen saturation in a pathological direction (lower limit value 96%) has also a greater clinical relevance in untrained or sick individuals.

Sports medicine confirmed an increase in carbon dioxide (CO_2) retention, with an elevation in CO_2 partial pressure in the blood with larger respiratory dead space volumes.

In fact, dead space-induced CO_2 retention while wearing a mask during exercise was also experimentally proven. The effects of a short aerobic exercise under N95 masks were tested on sixteen healthy volunteers. This determined a significantly increased in end-expiratory partial pressure of carbon dioxide ($PETCO_2$) of plus 8 mmHg. The increase in blood carbon dioxide (CO_2) in the mask wearers under maximum load was plus 14% CO_2 for surgical masks and plus 23% CO_2 for N95 masks, an effect that could have clinical relevance in the pre-diseased, elderly and children, as these values strongly approached the pathological range.

In an interesting endurance study with eight subjects (aged 19 to 66), the gas content for O_2 and CO_2 under the masks was determined before and after exercise. Even at rest, the oxygen availability under the masks was 13% lower than without the masks and the carbon dioxide (CO_2) concentration was 30 times higher. Under stress, the oxygen concentration (O_2) below the mask dropped significantly by a further 3.7%, while the carbon dioxide concentration (CO_2) increased significantly by a further 20%. Correspondingly, the oxygen saturation (SpO_2) of the test persons also decreased significantly from 97.6 to 92.1%. The drop in oxygen saturation value (SpO_2) to 92%, clearly below the normal limit of 96%, is to be classified as clinically relevant and detrimental to health.

These facts are an indication that the use of masks also triggers the effects described above leading to hypoxia and hypercapnia in sports. Accordingly, the WHO and Centres for Disease Control and Prevention (CDC) advise against wearing masks during physical exercise.

Increase in obesity risk

Another adverse effect of wearing mask is linked with an increase in obesity due to poor oxygenation.

Furthermore, mask wearing can also exacerbate obesity hypoventilation syndrome (OHS). This illness causes poor breathing in some people with obesity. It leads to lower oxygen and higher carbon dioxide levels in the blood. The exact cause of OHS is not known. It is believed that OHS results from a defect in the brain's control over breathing. Excess weight against the chest wall also makes it harder for the muscles to draw in a deep breath and to breathe quickly enough. This worsens the brain's breathing control. As a result, the blood contains too much carbon dioxide and not enough oxygen. Needless to remark that mask wearing would only make the issue worse.

 In conclusion, the German study:

"Is a Mask That Covers the Mouth and Nose Free from Undesirable Side Effects in Everyday Use and Free of Potential Hazards?" lists the main side effects caused by long-term mask wearing as follows:

Internal diseases	Psychiatric illness	Neurological Diseases
COPD	Claustrophobia	Migraines and Headache
Sleep Apnoea	Panic Disorder	Patients with intracranial Masses
Advanced renal failure	Personality Disorders	Epilepsy
Obesity	Dementia	**Dermatological Diseases**
Cardiopulmonary Dysfunction	Schizophrenia	Acne
Asthma	Helpless Patients	Atopic Irritation
Paediatric Diseases	Fixed and sedated Patients	
Respiratory Diseases	**ENT Diseases**	
Cardiopulmonary Diseases	Vocal Cord Disorders	
	Rhinitis and obstructive Diseases	
	Periodontitis and oral infections	

CHAPTER SIX

The expert's view

"The truth is like a lion: you do not have to defend it. Let it loose: it will defend itself." - St. Augustine

"The only thing necessary for the triumph of evil is for good men to do nothing." - Edmund Burke

This chapter describes in detail what one of the most prominent world experts has to say on masks and protection against aerosol viruses. His name is Stephen Petty. He is a qualified industrial hygienist in the USA with undergraduate and graduate degrees in chemical engineering and an MBA with training in the art of persuasion. He also is a Certified Safety Professional (C.S.P.) and a Professional Engineer -P.E. (Florida, Texas, Ohio, Kentucky, Pennsylvania, and West Virginia) with nine patents who has been working for 45 years in the field of health and safety. He taught as an adjunct Professor at Franklin University and taught Environmental and Earth Sciences. He spent his entire professional life trying to protect workers and the public from harm, ranging from anthrax to bio toxins. He has been disclosed in over 400 cases in respect to exposure control and PPE and he was serving as an expert witness in the Monsanto Roundup cases. Recently he testified in the State of Kentucky and, as a result of his testimony, the mask mandate was overturned state-wide.

Industrial hygiene is not well understood by many, especially the public and the media. Several so called 'experts' are talking about this subject even when this is not their field of expertise. Industrial hygiene is "the science and art devoted to the anticipation, recognition, evaluation and control of those environmental factors or stressors arising in or from the workplace, which may cause sickness, impaired health and well-being, or significant discomfort among workers or among the citizen of the community ". The core issue, in Petty's opinion, is that most people have heard of medical doctors, dentists and other professionals but they have not heard of industrial hygienists or industrial hygiene.

These exposure expert's occupation is to figure out and anticipate the reasons why people get sick and what might be hurting them. There are a lot of clinicians talking about this subject pretending to be knowledgeable on the matter when they are not. They may be perfectly talented individuals, but this is not their field. They pontificate on exposure and PPE and really do not have training in that dimension. It would be like to ask your dentist to perform heart surgery. In trials there are doctors talking about the disease whilst the industrial hygienists talk about exposure control. Most of the time doctors' statements are not based on facts and scientific data because that is not their background.

In the case of viruses in general and COVID in particular, Petty states that exposure is a function of three main parameters: time (the least we are exposed the better), concentration (the higher the concentration the higher the risk of disease) and distance (in general, the further we are from the source of illness the better).

In reality, there are three ways in which Stephen Petty proves, with no doubt, that masks cannot, and do not work. Moreover, the two meters (6') rule is not based on science but on the unhealthy congregation of politicians and technocrats; Scott Gottlieb, former FDA commissioner admitted in late 2021 that the US rule was simply made-up and had no basis in science.

In the first instance Mr. Petty states that if masks could work, we would expect for COVID cases to drop-in time, but they do not. In consulting statistics for any state and any country in the world it can be noticed that where people are indoors more, as in northern climates, the wintertime disease rates go up. Similarly, in warmer climates with air conditioning (e.g., southern climates), rate rise as people spend more times indoors. This has been a well understood industrial hygiene fact for over a hundred years; contaminants tend to concentrate indoors. The second factor he considers is based on epidemiology. He states that there have been many studies but probably the most relevant has been conducted in Denmark. Researchers looked at about ~6,000 people, ~3,000 with mask and ~3,000 without. Statistically, the authors found no difference in disease rates between the control and test groups. A similar study was done at schools in Florida and reaching the same conclusions. When he testified in the federal court in Michigan, in reference to a CDC study, he showed that almost all the research they cited suffered from two major flaws. The first one was that they did not have a control group not wearing masks to study the differences. If you do not have a control group how do you determine what makes a difference? The second aspect was the confusion created by too many overlapping factors happening at the same time such as air conditioning, social distancing, isolation and quarantine. In this way there was no way of knowing whether masking had any effect or otherwise. For Petty, in the past fifty years, the real solution has always been engineering control through ventilation, dilution or destruction of the hazards. Petty implemented those solutions in an actual school in 2020 (~700 autistic children) and he has worked with many districts to apply those measures in their buildings.

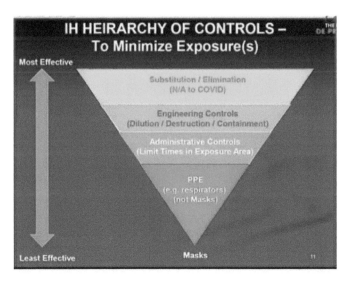

The hierarchy of controls is the underlining structure of those recommendations implemented to minimize exposure. This has been a fundamental concept in industrial hygiene since it was developed by the National Safety Council (NSC) in 1950. It lists and prioritizes the order of interventions in order to control people's exposure. The first measure is substitution or elimination and this does not really apply to COVID. It is only possible when hazardous material can be replaced by a less hazardous one. The next most effective action is either dilute, destroy or contain contaminants or hazards. Due to the fact that it is quite difficult to contain COVID, the remaining keys are dilution, destruction and administrative controls which entails to limit the time of stay in the spaces of contamination. Indoor spaces (rather than outdoor) are where you get the disease. Petty was very perplexed when the former Mayor of New York City, and many other heads of State decided to keep everybody indoors preventing people to go to the parks and to the beaches. The safest place to be is outside with maximum fresh air, not inside where contaminants can build up. The last, least effective and desirable way to protect people in this hierarchy of controls is PPE in the form of respirators. The bottom of the barrel for a respirator would be a N95 (FFP2). It is important to notice that surgical masks do not even fall on this list of controls and they are not considered PPE.

For Petty masks and respirators are always the least desirable option because they do not protect from infection, they are uncomfortable and people do not wear them properly. He considers individuals with facial hair and beards wearing mask a hilarious proposition in regard to infection prevention. The real solution is to get rid of the problem.

On the subject of masks Petty believes that OSHA is either misleading, at best, or dishonest at worst. This institution only recommends (not requires) readers (page 1 of the guidance) to wear a mask but on page six of their guidance states that "surgical masks are not respirators and do not provide the same level of protection to workers as properly fitted respirators. Cloth face coverings are also not acceptable substitutes for respirators." This is a tacit admission masks or facial covering do not work and a contradiction with Industrial Hygiene standard of care illustrated by the Hierarchy of Controls. If someone would recommend in court that people being exposed to asbestos fibers should be protected by wearing a mask, they would probably lose all their credentials. It is not that OSHA directors are not smart; they are just dishonest or at best disingenuous. CDC is really no better: on their website they state that masks do not provide the wearer with a reliable level of protection from inhaling smaller airborne powder coats and they are not to be considered respiratory protection. In any surgical mask container, we find similar affirmations in one form or another. The consequent logical question to ask would then be: "why are we required to wear them?"

The third point that Petty makes is based on micro perspectives. What the science is really suggesting is that the matter of concern are aerosols particles. The initial recommendations at the start of the pandemic were the repeating "ad nauseam" of the three words "surfaces, surfaces, surfaces" then they moved to "droplets, droplets, droplets" and then they started to consider some science and went "ooh, maybe, aerosols, aerosols, aerosols" when this should have been the first and only approach.

In his experience in working with silica and asbestos the spectrum of size of the particles is the most important aspect. The definitions specify that aerosols are less than 5 microns in size whilst droplets are between 5 to 10 microns. Another definition speaks about "respirable particles" always being five microns or less. They are called "respirable" because they go deep in the lungs and they can stay suspended for hours and days in our indoor environments. The smallest specks cause most concern because they move deeply into the lungs whereas the larger droplets either fall to the ground or they are halted by the mucous tissues.

There has been great disinformation about COVID being a droplet. In reality in coronavirus over 99.9% of the particles are aerosols. If OSHA, CDC and any other public health agency would admit that the primary mechanism of exposure is aerosols, masks and the six-foot rule would collapse. This is why they're very nervous about the term aerosol, because that also means that the entire world was exposed to the virus, with virtually no protection, for the past two years.

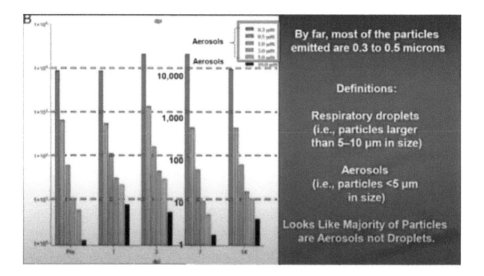

A National Academy of Sciences press article by Edwards, et al reporting on a study conducted on monkeys and the size of breathing particles pre-infection and after infection. The findings clearly show that the higher and dominant percentage of particles are aerosols, not droplets.

Transmission through inhalation of small aerosol particles is an important and significant mode of transmission of COVID. The gravity of the problem has been emphasized also by an editorial in the journal "Nature".

Numerous studies have demonstrated that aerosols produced through breathing, talking and singing are concentrated close to the infected person, remain in the air, are viable for long periods of time and travel long distances within a room and sometimes further.

Gathering in indoor spaces without adequate ventilation places individuals at particular risk.

The CDC recognizes inhalation as a route of exposure that should be controlled to protect against COVID but most guidance and recommendations do not address inhalation exposure to small aerosol particles.

On February 22nd 2022 eight industrial hygienists wrote to CDC, Dr. Fauci and the White House regarding this aerosol issue. Still the CDC continues to use outdated confusing terms such as "respiratory droplets" to describe both larger propelled droplets and the smaller inhalable aerosol particles. It also confuses matters with "airborne transmission" to indicate inhalation exposure exclusively at long distances and does not consider inhalation exposure via the same aerosol at short distances. Their recommendations do not include the control measures necessary for protecting the public and the workers from inhalation exposure to SARS-COVID2 when aerosol is the kingpin word that renders masks and the two meters rule essentially meaningless.

Even the National academies' notes on "airborne transmission" focuses on route of exposure via touch, large droplets sprayed onto the body and inhalation of small aerosol particles.

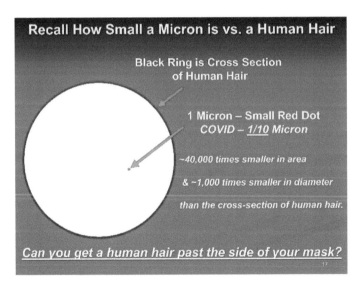

In order to understand in practice the size of COVID we can use this picture which compares the different dimensions of particles compared to a human hair. A micron is the red dot which is 4 000 times smaller than a human hair. The virus can be as small as a tenth of a micron in terms of size. Petty often asks people if they think it would be possible to slide a human hair by the side of their mask especially below the eyes.

Everybody obviously says yes. This is consequently and obviously a super freeway for a virus to come and go. Any argument contradicting this fact, in Petty's opinion is mere nonsense. What happens with the virus becomes self-explanatory.

Another study is based on Stokes law and calculates, giving its density, how fast a particle falls five feet (which would be similar to the distance from somebody's mouth to the floor).

SMALL PARTICLES TAKE A LONG TIME TO FALL FIVE FEET IN STILL AIR

Aerosols Fall Slowly: 0.03 to 59 days

Particle Size (µm)	Time to Fall 5' (days)	Type of Particle
0.09	58.9	COVID
0.12	46.4	
0.2	16.7	Aerosol
1	0.67	
5	0.027	

COVID-19 Fall Very Slowly: Up to 46.4 to 58.9 days

Stokes' Law - assumes still air; in moving air times would be even longer.

Droplets of 10- 25-100 microns fall to the ground in about one minute - nine minutes - one hour in relation to their size. Particles between 0.5 microns to a tenth of a micron need between one and 59 days.

The virus is around 0.1 to 0.3 microns so these particles stay suspended in still air from seven to fifty days. If the ventilation in the room is poor the virus particles also accumulate. We could be shopping in a supermarket which has been visited by a sick person few days earlier and the virus is still floating around.

Nobody has been provided by the Creator with a COVID meter on the chest or in the head. If someone has been sick in the office yesterday or last week nobody has a way of knowing whether the particles are still there or not.

These calculations are also done in still air. But imagine what happens to particles of dust (25 microns) moving and dancing in the sunlight. This happens with the virus too, even if you cannot see them, because the particles are too small to be visible. This explains why masks and the six feet rule has no meaning. Petty always gets asked if masks have zero effectiveness. He replies with another question:" Can a mosquito go through a chain-link fence wall?"

Again, Petty thinks that the only solutions from an industrial hygiene standpoint are dilution, ventilation and destruction. This has been determined by the USA National Safety Council in 1950, seventy years ago. Masks did not make these recommendations void or change in any way the reality of science. By definition a mask cannot be sealed and cannot offer protection.

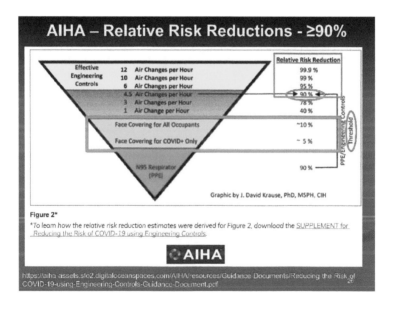

Some people say: "Well, masks might do a little bit of good." Industrial hygiene does not look at solutions that to do a little bit of good. Masks might help 1% of the people but not the public in general. Implemented measures must provide at least a 90% relative reduction.

How would anyone feel if a regulator walked in a work place and said to asbestos workers: "Let's put you in a mask. It might save 1% of you from asbestosis but the other 99% will get it". That technician would lose all licenses.

By the way asbestos fiber, on average, is 50 times larger than coronavirus particles. So, why in the world would someone take a 1% solution when what is needed is a 90%? With implementing ventilation, destruction and filtration it is possible to meet that 90% requirement.

Petty says that he would not even use an N95 for asbestos workers. One of the issues with masks is that they do not provide a sufficient seal against aerosols They are a freeway for anything to come and go. To say that it will protect others even if it does not protect you or vice versa is the same as stating that a bird can fly in through an open window but not fly out from the same.

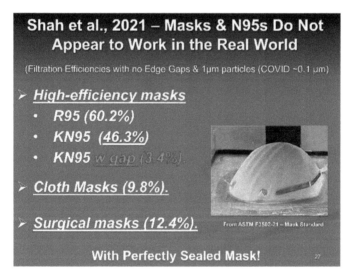

In a study by Shaw at al. that shows no satisfactory results even for an N95 when this is glued onto a board. This is how most of these studies are done. They literally glue the mask onto a mannequin or a board. But does anyone glue a mask on their face? Of course not. When the mask is glued to the board it shows a 46% effectiveness. Having just one gap decreases the effectiveness to 3%. Imagine what could be the case in the real world.

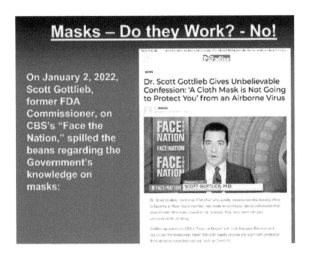

On January 2nd 2022 Scott Godly, a FDA commissioner spilled the beans. He basically declared that masks do not work. Finally, on January 14th of 2022, the CDC admitted the same. In two years, the CDC scientific guidance changed opinion many times and had several 180 degree turns: masks do not work, masks work, masks do not work. No science does that.

Petty also said that, in February 2022 he wrote a letter to the CDC complaining about this aspect. His petition was disregarded and the White House, along with some specialists, said, instead, that they wanted to put children in N95 masks linking the public to the manufacturers' websites for reference. One of those was 3M; what does 3M state? That N95 are "not designated to be used by children"! One of the consequences in this irresponsible behaviour is in the failure to adhere to respiratory protection standards which consists in a long list of requirements. It is not possible to ask someone to wear a N95 mask and not incur in many liabilities.

Failure to fit test a mask, lack of certainty that individuals are medically cleared to wear one or that a tailored training on how to wear and replace them has been planned could result in legal actions against the employer.

In UK, by law, the employer should undertake individual risk assessments on each and every employee to comply with the law. I personally do not know anyone that had been specifically and individually assessed prior to wear masks and PPE.

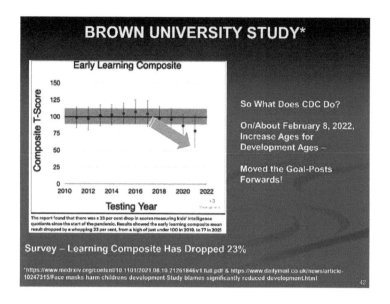

BROWN UNIVERSITY STUDY*

Early Learning Composite

So What Does CDC Do?

On/About February 8, 2022,
Increase Ages for
Development Ages –

Moved the Goal-Posts
Forwards!

The report found that there was a 23 per cent drop in scores measuring kids' intelligence quotients since the start of the pandemic. Results showed the early learning composite mean result dropped by a whopping 23 per cent, from a high of just under 100 in 2019, to 77 in 2021

Survey – Learning Composite Has Dropped 23%

*https://www.medrxiv.org/content/10.1101/2021.08.10.21261846v1.full.pdf & https://www.dailymail.co.uk/news/article-10247315/Face-masks-harm-childrens-development-Study-blames-significantly-reduced-development.html

Lot of damage has also been done to children through mask mandates in schools. Recent data show impairment both for reading and for mathematics and a loss in performance between 12 and 15% depending on the grade level. Results are even worse for minorities. In a study, Brown University determined that children born during COVID and wearing masks showed a 23% reduction in development. The CDC strategy to solve the issue was puzzling.

On the 8th of February 2022 they changed a 18 year old criteria for child development and just moved the goal post. Instead of admitting that mask wearing was causing enormous damage they extended the performance standards for children from 24 months to 30.

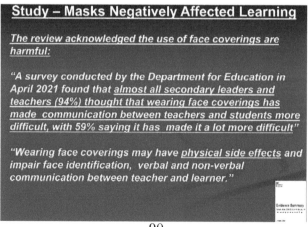

Study – Masks Negatively Affected Learning

The review acknowledged the use of face coverings are harmful:

"A survey conducted by the Department for Education in April 2021 found that almost all secondary leaders and teachers (94%) thought that wearing face coverings has made communication between teachers and students more difficult, with 59% saying it has made it a lot more difficult"

"Wearing face coverings may have physical side effects and impair face identification, verbal and non-verbal communication between teacher and learner."

Similarly, the England Department of Education noted that 94% of the teachers indicated that wearing face coverings had made communication more difficult and 59% said much more difficult. Lenski and other authors looked at 12,126 papers on masking, further reduced to 109 qualitative and 49 quantitative studies. This research showed 27 adverse effects they could quantitate including five specifically for children. In conclusion, Petty's closing statement is that masks cannot be a solution to a virus, any virus. He also declared that despite having given six national podcasts statements since the beginning of the pandemic, still available online and having spent almost a half a million of his own time and money building a studio and putting out a further 20 podcasts (https://rumble.com/c/PettyPodcasts) summarising the main points of his argument, complete with web URLs and detailed references.

ENGINEERING CONTROLS

From an IH Perspective, Engineering Controls:

➤ **Fresh Air**

➤ **Filtration**

➤ **Destruction.**

Have and Always Will be our Best Solutions.

In the Meantime – Quit Harming Our Children with Ineffective and Harmful Masks and Respirators.

He states that the solution has been for ~70 years, and will be for the foreseeable future, Engineering Controls of Dilution, Filtration and Destruction.

It seems that officials and government do not wish to act on factual and scientific data.

CHAPTER SEVEN

Masks: emotional and psychological harm

"If God would judge that mask wearing is good for us, She would provide us with one at birth." – Lucia Bruno

In the previous chapter we explored the more palpable and measurable physical harms provoked by mask wearing.

The social, sociological, relational and psychological hazards are somehow more difficult to determine from a quantitative perspective. Nonetheless, they are far from being less damaging and disturbing. As follows the reader can look into some of the more obvious effects on this subject.

SOCIAL AND SOCIOLOGICAL SIDE EFFECTS AND DANGERS

Impaired communication

Clear communication is a vital requirement in any setting and it is even more important in health services, work places and schools where it is a prerequisite for the delivering of appropriate support and assistance, effective healthcare and to minimise mistakes and misunderstanding that can cost lives. Dampened speech and the inability to recognise non-verbal signals, makes masks a significant impediment in correct information sharing. This obstacle has the effect of potentially impairing the ability to understand clinical problems, recommended therapeutic interventions, operational instructions and correctly comprehending teachers input. Foreigners, minorities and those with hearing impairment who often rely on lip-reading, will suffer the most. In this country, there are approximately 11 million people with a hearing loss which makes it the second most common disability in the UK.

However, being an invisible disability, it very often goes unnoticed, making it easier for those living with this impairment to be ignored or forgotten. Statistics tell us that 1 in 6 people in the UK adult population is affected by hearing loss, 8 million of these are aged 60 and over, 6.7 million could benefit from hearing aids but only about 2 million people use them, about 900,000 people are severely or profoundly deaf. Those impacted by this mask-induced communication problem will have to undergo daily distress with, at times, devastating consequences.

The results of a Chilean study in health care also show that masks act like an acoustic filter and provoke excessively loud speech. This causes voice disorders. The increased volume of speech also contributes to increased aerosol production by the mask wearer. These experimental data are highly relevant.

Moreover, mask wearers are prevented from interacting normally in everyday life due to impaired clarity of speech, which tempts them to get closer to each other.

This results in a distorted prioritisation in the general public, which counteracts the recommended measures associated with the COVID-19 pandemic. The WHO prioritises social distancing and hand hygiene with moderate evidence and recommends wearing a mask with weak evidence, especially in situations where individuals are unable to maintain a physical distance of at least 1 metre.

The disruption of non-verbal communication due to the loss of facial expression recognition under the mask can increase feelings of insecurity, discouragement and numbness as well as isolation, which can be extremely stressful for the mentally and hearing-impaired.

On this subject I can describe my experience in one of this year's University lessons. The lecturer was constantly wearing a FFP3 mask and would also ask us to wear a surgical one. All I can remember about that module is "mumble, burble, babble and garble". This would happen during her speech, every time someone was asking questions or when the teacher was answering them. After a while the students got tired of keeping asking to repeat and just regarded the fact as one of the many inconveniences of the pandemic and decided to only rely on the written handouts. Obviously, attending lessons became of little use until the teacher finally stopped with the requirement. This was even more distressing for me and the other foreign students. We had not realised how much we were relying on lip reading for our comprehension of spoken words.

Experts point out that masks disrupt the basics of human communication (verbal and nonverbal). The limited facial recognition caused by masks leads to a suppression of emotional signals. Masks, therefore, disrupt social interaction, erasing the positive effect of smiles and laughter but at the same time greatly increasing the likelihood of misunderstandings because negative emotions are also less evident under masks.

A decrease in empathy perception through mask use with disruption of the doctor–patient relationship has already been scientifically proven on the basis of a randomised study. In this, the Consultation Empathy Care Measurement, the Patient Enablement Instrument (PEI) score and a Satisfaction Rating Scale were assessed in 1030 patients. The 516 doctors, who wore masks throughout, conveyed reduced empathy towards the patients and, thus, nullified the positive health-promoting effects of a dynamic relationship. These results demonstrate a disruption of interpersonal interaction and relationship dynamics caused by masks.

The WHO guidance on the use of masks in children in the community, published in August 2020, points out that the benefits of mask use in children must be weighed up against the potential harms, including social and communicational concerns.

Fears that widespread pandemic measures will lead to dysfunctional social life with degraded social, cultural and psychological interactions have also

Deprivation of freedom and related consequences

We have determined that mask wearing causes, amongst other things an impaired field of vision mostly related to the ground and obstacles on the ground. Furthermore, it inhibits the execution of habitual actions such as eating, drinking, touching, scratching and cleaning the otherwise normally uncovered part of the face. This hinderance is consciously and subconsciously perceived as a permanent disturbance, obstruction and restriction. Wearing masks, consequently, entails a feeling of deprivation of freedom and loss of autonomy and self-determination, which can lead to suppressed anger and subconscious constant distraction, especially as the wearing of masks is mostly dictated and ordered by others.

These perceived interferences on integrity, self-determination and autonomy, coupled with discomfort, often contribute to substantial disturbance and may ultimately be combined with physiologically mask-related decline in psycho-motor abilities, reduced responsiveness and an overall impaired cognitive performance. This also leads to misjudging situations as well as delayed, incorrect and inappropriate behaviour and a decline in the overall effectiveness of the mask wearer.

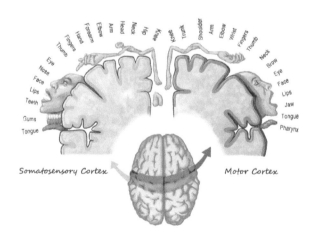

A fact very often disregarded by science is that the head and face are significant for well-being due to their large representation in the sensitive cerebral cortex (homunculus). In this document there is not enough space to explore the massive implication of this phenomenon in human physiology and behaviour but in short the cortical homunculus, or "cortex man," illustrates the concept of a representation of the body lying within the brain. The amount of cortex devoted to any given body region is not proportional to that body region's surface area or volume, but rather to how richly innervated that region is. Areas of the body with more complex and/or more numerous sensory or motor connections are represented as larger in the homunculus, while those with less complex and/or less numerous connections are represented as smaller.

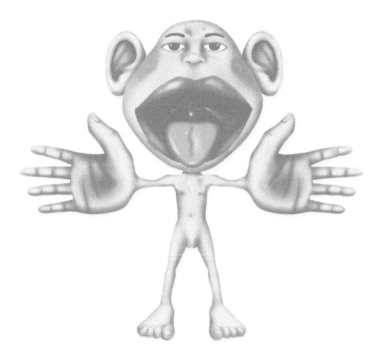

The resulting image is that of a distorted human body, with disproportionately huge hands, lips, and face. As a consequence, what affects the human face has a greater effect on our brain than on other parts of the body. This has been known and applied for millennia in yoga in general and in Yoga Nidra in particular. Yoga Nidra has been able to access and resolve many psychological and unconscious issues simply focusing on the systematic physical relaxation of the body by default influencing the corresponding brain areas. Needless to say, the relaxation concentrates the most and specifically on the brain areas represented as larger in the homunculus.

According to studies and surveys, masks also frequently cause anxiety and psycho-vegetative stress reactions in children as well as in adults, with an increase in psychosomatic and stress-related illnesses, depressive self-experience, reduced participation, social withdrawal and lowered health-related self-care. Over 50% of the mask wearers studied had at least mild depressive feelings.

Additional fear-inducing and often exaggerated media coverage can further intensify this. A recent retrospective analysis of the official media in the context of the 2014 Ebola epidemic showed a scientific truth content of only 38% of all publicly circulated information.

Researchers classified a total of 28% of the information as provocative and polarising and 42% as exaggerating risks. In addition, 72% of the media content aimed to stir up health-related negative feelings. The feeling of fear, combined with insecurity and the primal human need to belong, causes a social dynamic that seems critical from a medical and scientific point of view.

The mask, which originally served a purely hygienic purpose, has been transformed into a symbol of conformity and pseudo-solidarity. The WHO, for example, lists the advantages of the use of masks by healthy people in public to include:

"a potentially reduced stigmatisation of mask wearers, a sense of contribution to preventing the spread of the virus and a reminder to comply with other measures."

Psychiatric Side Effects and Dangers

As explained earlier, masks can cause increased rebreathing with an accumulation of carbon dioxide in the wearer due to increased dead space volume, with often statistically significant measurable elevated blood carbon dioxide (CO_2) levels in the sufferers. Those changes that lead to hypercapnia are known to trigger panic attacks. This makes the significantly measurable increase in CO_2 caused by wearing a mask clinically relevant.

Interestingly, breath provocation tests by inhaling CO_2 are used to differentiate anxiety states in panic disorders and premenstrual dysphoria from other psychiatric clinical illnesses. Absolute concentrations of 5% CO_2 are already sufficient to trigger panic reactions within 15–16 minutes considering that the normal exhaled air content of CO_2 is about 4%.

From experimental studies on masked subjects, it is obvious that concentration changes in the respiratory gases with values above 4% could occur whilst rebreathing and during prolonged mask use.

This is even more important if we consider that the activation of the locus coeruleus by CO_2 generates panic reactions and several other disturbing adverse reactions.

The locus coeruleus (LC), a small brainstem nucleus, is the primary source of the neuromodulator norepinephrine (NE) in the brain. Norepinephrine (NE) is one of the four main neuromodulators in the brain, exerting widespread influence over almost all cortical and subcortical brain regions. Neurons in the locus coeruleus (LC) release NE to regulate baseline arousal and to facilitate a variety of sensory-motor and behavioural functions. Dysfunction in the LC-NE system has been implicated in the aetiology of ADHD, schizophrenia, anxiety, stress and depression, as well as in the cognitive decline observed in ageing and Alzheimer's disease.

From the physiological, neurological and psychological side effects and dangers described above, additional problems can be derived for the use of masks in psychiatric cases. People undergoing treatment for dementia, paranoid schizophrenia, personality disorders, anxiety and panic disorders with claustrophobic components, are difficult to reconcile with a mask requirement, because even small increases in CO_2 can cause and intensify those diseases.

According to a psychiatric study, patients with moderate to severe dementia have no understanding of COVID-19 protection measures and have to be persuaded to wear masks constantly.

According to a comparative study, patients with schizophrenia have a lower acceptance of mask-wearing (54.9% agreement) than ordinary patients (61.6%). The extent to which mask-wearing can lead to an exacerbation of schizophrenia symptoms has not yet been researched in detail.

When wearing masks, confusion, impaired thinking, disorientation and in some cases a decrease in maximum speed and reaction time were observed. In mental health treatment, psychotropic drugs reduce psycho-motor functions in psychiatric patients. This can become clinically relevant especially with regard to the further reduced ability to react and the additional increased susceptibility to accidents of such patients when wearing masks.

In order to avoid an unintentional CO_2-triggered anaesthesia, medically sedated patients, without the possibility of continuous monitoring, should not be masked according to the criteria of the Centre for Disease Control and Prevention, (CDC). This is because of the possible CO_2 retention described above, as there is a risk of unconsciousness, aspiration and asphyxia.

Other studies showed that the psychological and physical effects of the masks can lead to an additional reduction in work attendance via increased feelings of fatigue, dissatisfaction and anxiety.

Finally, a disproportionately high number of attendees at hospitals and GP practices will display existing mental health problems. Many people already tormented by recurrent panic attacks, involving catastrophic thoughts of imminent death and feelings of breathlessness, will find masks very difficult to tolerate. Similarly, those suffering obsessive-compulsive fears about the prospect of contamination, or severe health anxieties, will have their emotional difficulties intensified by regular mask wearing.

It is a common misconception that a face covering will provide reassurance - on the contrary, habitual wearing will prolong their fears. Many people on the autistic spectrum will be distressed by the expectation and (overt and covert) pressure to wear a mask.

Social and Occupational Medicine Side Effects and Hazards

In work and school settings, in addition to mask-specific complaints such as a feeling of heat, dampness, shortness of breath and headache, various physiological phenomena were documented, such as the significant increase in heart and respiratory rate, the impairment of lung function parameters, the decrease in cardiopulmonary capacity as well as changes in oxygen and carbon dioxide that was measured in the blood of the individuals. The significant changes were measurable after only a few minutes of wearing a mask and in some cases reached magnitudes of minus 13% of O_2 and a 30-fold increase in CO_2 concentration of the inhaled air under masks. The changes observed were not only statistically significant, but also clinically relevant; the subjects also showed pathological oxygen saturation after exposure to masks.

Shortness of breath during light exertion (6 min walking) under surgical masks has been recorded with statistical significance in forty four healthy subjects in a prospective experimental intervention study.

Wearing masks over a longer period of time consequently led to physiological and psychological impairments in other studies and, thus, reduced work performance. In experiments on respiratory-protective equipment, an increase in the dead space volume of 350 ml leads to a reduction in the possible performance time of approximately minus 19%, and a decrease in breathing comfort of minus18%.

In addition, the time spent working and the flow of work is interrupted and reduced by putting on and taking off the masks and changing them. The reduced work performance has been recorded in the literature found, as described above, but has not been quantified further in detail.

Other studies described subjective reduced work performance and mask-related impairments in users. Objectively, another study determined that wearing N95 masks results in hypooxygenemia and hypercapnia which reduce working efficiency and the ability to make correct decision. A further study confirmed that chronic hypoxia-hypercapnia influences and debilitates cognitive functions. The abstract stated that chronic obstructive pulmonary disease (COPD), a slowly progressive lung disease, results in several complications, including cognitive dysfunction. In a circular way, it has also been confirmed that chronic hypoxia-hypercapnia hugely contributes to the development of COPD.

In brief, cognitive impairment is strongly related to combinations of chronic hypoxia and hypercapnia which are exacerbated by wearing masks.

Due to the relatively larger representation in the sensitive cerebral cortex (homunculus), the temperature sensation in the face is more decisive for the feeling of well-being than other body regions. The perception of discomfort when wearing a mask can, thus, be intensified. In seven of eight studies, a combined occurrence of the physical variable "temperature rise under the mask" and the symptom "respiratory impairment" caused a mutual significantly measured occurrence in 88% of cases. It was also detected a combined occurrence of significantly measured temperature rise under the mask and significant measurement of fatigue in 50% of the relevant primary studies. These clustered association of temperature rise with symptoms of respiratory impairment and fatigue suggests a clinical relevance of the detected temperature rise under masks. In the worst-case scenario, the effects mentioned can reinforce each other and lead to decompensation, especially in the presence of COPD, heart failure and respiratory insufficiency.

The sum of the disturbances and discomforts that can be caused by a mask also contributes to distraction. These, in conjunction with a decrease in psycho-motor skills, reduced responsiveness and overall impaired cognitive performance (all of which are pathophysiological effects of wearing a mask) can lead to a failure to recognise hazards and, thus, to accidents or avoidable errors at work.

Of particular note here are mask-induced lethargy, impaired thinking and concentration problems as measured by a Likert scale. Accordingly, occupational health regulations act against such scenarios. For example, the German Industrial Accident Insurance (DGUV) has precise and extensive regulations for respiratory protective equipment where they document the limitation of wearing time, levels of work intensity and several other obligations.

The standards and norms prescribed in many countries regarding different types of masks to protect their workers are also significant from an occupational health point of view. In Germany there are very strict safety specifications for masks compared to other countries. These specify the requirements for the protection of the wearer. All these standards and the accompanying certification procedures were increasingly relaxed with the introduction of mandatory masks for the general public. This meant that non-certified masks such as community masks were also used on a large scale in work and school settings and for longer periods during the pandemic.

Most recently, in October 2020, the German Social Accident Insurance (DGUV) recommended the same usage time limits for community masks as for filtering half masks, namely, a maximum of three shifts of 120 minutes per day with recovery breaks of 30 minutes in between. In Germany, FFP2 (N95) masks must be worn for 75 minutes, followed by a 30-minute break. An additional suitability examination by specialised physicians is also obligatory and stipulated for occupationally used masks.

None of those scientifically lead and sensible measures were implemented in UK.

Relational Harm

Along with headaches, trouble breathing, cardio-pulmonary stress, discomfort, and cognitive impairment, another significant realm of harms caused by masks is relational.

A study published in 1996 by the journal "Perceptual and Motor Skills" investigated how smiles, hidden by masks, affect people's perceptions of other people. The study involved a sample of 330 Brazilian college students who were shown photos of people who were smiling and not smiling. Consistent with earlier research, documented by the authors, the study found, for example "a powerful effect of facial expression on person perception.", smiling people were perceived as kinder, more attractive, more sympathetic, more sincere, more sociable, and more competent.

As explained by a 2009 paper in the "American Journal of Infection Control", people "cannot see most facial expressions of a person wearing a mask," and this can impede social bonding "because it obscures an important nonverbal mode of communication."

A study published in 2008 by the journal "Neuropsychologia" evaluated the memory and brain activity of eighteen young adults who were shown pictures and names of people with smiling and neutral faces. The study found that the subjects remembered the names of 59.0% of the smiling faces and 46.8% of the neutral faces.

The smiling faces activated certain regions of the subjects' brains more fully than the neutral faces proving that "rewarding social signals from a smiling face can enhance relational memory."

In 2020, a trade journal called the "Hearing Review" published a laboratory study of communication impediments caused by N95 and surgical masks.

The study and other research conducted by the authors showed that a "cornerstone of patient safety and quality healthcare is effective communication which allows patients to participate fully in their care."

Healthcare is "often being delivered in settings which are extremely noisy and distracting - repleted with alarms beeping and ongoing competing conversations between patients and providers."

"Our findings were not unexpected but were unsettling. Masks filtered out the high frequencies (2000–7000 Hz) spoken by the wearer, with the decibel (dB) level of attenuation ranging from 3 to 4 dB for a simple medical mask and close to 12 dB for the N95 masks."

For reference, a reduction of 10 dBs amounts to halving the loudness of a sound.

"In short, the speech quality degradation, in combination with room noise/reverberation and the absence of visual cues, renders speech close to unintelligible for many."

A study published in 2020 by the "Journal of Laryngology & Otology" found the following about communication impediments caused by using N95 surgical masks with face shields: "Use of personal protective equipment (PPE) significantly impairs speech perception."

The volume at which people could recognise certain two-syllable words spoken by someone wearing a N95 mask and a face shield must increase by 12.4 decibels to be equivalent to someone speaking without PPE. This amounts to a doubling in loudness.

Even at 40 decibels above the speech reception threshold, the ability of people to recognise certain words spoken by someone wearing a N95 mask and a face shield declined by 7%. "Our study was performed in a sound-treated audiology setting in order to standardise the environment for quantitative assessment. However, most conversations in the healthcare setting occur in the scenario of significant ambient noise. This may further impair speech perception and intelligibility."

"The role of cues obtained from lip reading and facial expressions in the perception of speech cannot be ignored. These might have a negligible role in a normal hearing individual and in a quiet environment, but not for those with hearing impairment and in the presence of background noise."

A study published in 2021 by the journal "Frontiers in Psychology" measured the ability of 119 people to sense the emotions of people who were masked. The study and other research conducted by the authors showed that: "facial movements and situational cues are crucial when interacting with others"; "a mask obstructing a face limits the ability of people of all ages to infer emotions expressed by facial features"; "the difficulties associated with the mask's use are significantly pronounced in children aged between 3 and 5 years old"; "sensitivity to facial emotion movements is fundamental to children's emotional processing and social competence"; "early childhood is considered a critical period for the development of understanding emotions and emotion processing" and "young children's future social abilities should be monitored to assess the true impact of the use of masks."

Human beings, and especially children, are highly social creatures. Masks stifle that by interfering with bonding and communication, which are essential to people's mental health, physical health, and productivity.

Because association does not prove causation, it is impossible to empirically determine if widespread masking has played a role in the accompanying surges of depression and anxiety among youth, suicides among teens and young adults, and drug overdoses among people of all ages. But given the effects of masks on relationships, it would be mindless and irresponsible to ignore or dismiss this possibility.

Unfortunately, while face coverings are disappearing from many spheres of daily life, they stubbornly remain evident in healthcare settings, where they are evolving into an integral part of the uniform. Doctors, nurses and allied-health professionals are becoming culturally wedded to masks, where, despite the absence of robust evidence to support their infection control benefits, they identify people as part of the team fighting against a virus, "working together to beat the enemy". Service users and their relatives are coerced into joining this war by the requirement to wear a face covering, a symbol that distinguishes ally from foe.

This cultural descent into ubiquitous masks in hospitals and health centres is hugely concerning. In addition to the specific harms associated with them, this ideological trend ignores a fundamental principle: a positive relationship between professional and patient is an essential ingredient of a healing environment. Warmth, empathy, trust and openness, key elements of a therapeutic relationship, are more difficult to demonstrate when access to facial expressions is impeded.

Many psychological therapy sessions are undertaken in hospitals and GP practices, and, throughout the pandemic, these have often been conducted in environments that require both patient and practitioner to wear a mask. Although little research has been done on the impact of COVID restrictions on the effectiveness of specialist talking therapy, the limited human connection between two faceless people is likely to be especially problematic, compromising the usefulness of these interventions for people struggling with emotional difficulties.

But the therapeutic damage associated with masks is not limited to the realm of specialist psychological interventions. Human connection is the bedrock of the healing process.

As a consequence of the often obstructed relationships resulting from masked characters, service users of all kinds will experience sub-optimal care: the confused, hard-of-hearing elderly person with memory loss; the apprehensive cancer patient receiving test results; the distressed teenager contemplating deliberate self-harm; and the frightened child in acute pain. Humane healthcare, delivered with demonstrable warmth and compassion, will always be more effective than the robotic version delivered by a faceless professional hidden behind a veneer of sterility.

In the words of one enlightened GP, it's time to "put the patient first again" by ditching the mask in healthcare settings.

Re-traumatising those with histories of abuse

Another group of people who will be affected by mask wearing in healthcare settings are those who have suffered historical sexual and physical abuse. Many of these victims will be re-traumatised by the requirement to wear face masks, from the somatic sensation of material covering the nose and mouth. Simply the sight of masked people can trigger disturbing memories ("flashbacks") of assault and degradation. To make matters worse, exercising one's legal right to go without a face covering is likely to attract harassment and victimisation, particularly when in hospitals and other health-related venues. Here just one of the many anonymous testimonials:

"Eleven years ago I was attacked; grabbed from behind by a man holding an arm over my nose and mouth to silence my scream, I was then held at knifepoint for hours on my kitchen floor. This is why I have never worn a mask, it's too much for me to have my mouth and nose covered in this way. I shouldn't have to explain this to anyone (I never have) but I almost feel like I have to justify why I won't and can't comply with the mask rules."

CHAPTER EIGHT

Masks: environmental harm

"Breath is sacred. It animates our body, it gives force and power to our words, chants and songs, and it enables us to purify ourselves and our cells. It is powerful. It gives meaning and language, it can carry great wisdom (or foolishness) and it can store power or send it outwards." – Ravenari

In this chapter I will bring my mother back in. She is an unintended environmental warrior, by misadventure rather than out of a political choice. Mostly this is due to her culture and upbringing in which 'waste' and 'sin' are somehow synonymous. In the seventies we went to live in the countryside in a house with a hectare of land. Very little was going into the trash bin. We were 90% self-sufficient food wise and everything was painstakingly reused and recycled. Food leftovers were going to the goat and the chickens or otherwise in the compost heap, paper and cardboard were disposed on the latter or used to light the fireplace, water was coming from a hundred metre deep well which was making the need for plastic bottles totally redundant, I cannot remember a can of coke (or any other soda for that matter) arriving in the household at any given time.

The little that still had to be disposed was religiously flattened, divided into categories and carried to the local recycling area. My dad was doing his part re-routing water and electric pipes not to disturb moles underground pathways and dwellings. This family 'modus operandi' influenced my life and my way of doing architecture when I run my project management company. The buildings we were renovating in South of Italy had collection of water from the roofs, recycling of grey water for irrigation, solar panels for hot water and reed sewage treatment. Negligible amounts of matter and energy was going in or out of the buildings.

You can only imagine what my mother and I think about the mask disposal disgrace and the related environmental disaster of the past two years. Even before 2020, looking at the way NHS ruminates and pontificates about environmental issues whilst nobody, from top to bottom, does anything at all on the practical level and on a daily basis to actually pursue this ideal, would and still makes me furious. At work, I have two self-appointed tasks, the first is to remove any recyclable item from the trash bin and move them to the purposely allocated one which lives just next to it. The second is to become utterly hysterical when my colleagues run the dishwasher to only clean a single cup. I am not exaggerating, it happens at least once for every shift I work.

I also would like to mention that the first energetic lesson during my architecture university studies was that to transform valuable sources of energy such as electricity into mechanical power is a scientifically proven nonsense. The second one was that transforming one source of energy into another provokes immense waste of power at any given passage. This, on the practical level, means that it is reasonable for electricity to be produced with hydroelectric energy or to be derived from fossil fuels but it is wasteful to use the resulting precious electrical energy to retransform it in thermic energy to cook meals or in mechanical energy to move cars around.

Does any of the modern environmentalists know that the electricity you use for your car is mostly made with fossil fuels and that you need enormous amount of it?

Those basic principles are totally reversed and disregarded by the contorted logic of the so-called environmental movement. I am an ecologically very active and thoughtful individual but to use coal to produce electricity and then electricity to produce mechanical energy is still a no-no for me. And I do not even wish to go into other issues such as children abused to mine cobalt and lithium to be used in batteries for electric cars in a modern slavery fashion or the fact that the entire world production of these elements would never be sufficient to even cover the annual need of one single country or that those batteries have a life span of 7 to 10 years.

Going back to masks, the WHO estimates, at present, a demand of about 100 million masks per month and their global production will continue to increase. If even 1% of the masks are not disposed properly, and this is just wishful thinking, the result would be one million face masks per month dispersed in the environment.

Considering that the weight of each mask is about 4 grams, this would result in the dispersion of over 48000 kilograms of plastic a year.

A recent working paper by the Plastic Waste Innovation Hub at University College London has put the current domestic demand for the UK at 24.7 billion masks a year.

Due to the chemical composition of disposable surgical masks containing polymers such as polypropylene, polyurethane, polyacrylonitrile, polystyrene, polycarbonate, polyethylene and polyester the logical consequence is an increased global challenge from an environmental point of view, especially outside Europe where the absence of recycling and disposal strategies is more problematic. Single use polymers have been identified as a significant source of pollution of all water cycles from river sources to the marine environment.

A significant health hazard factor is also constituted by mask waste in the form of microplastics after decomposition into the food chain. Furthermore, contaminated disposable mask waste represents a widespread medium for microbes (protozoa, bacteria, viruses, fungi) in terms of invasive pathogens which are present in sufficient concentration and quantity to cause disease in susceptible hosts. Consequently, improper disposal of face masks has the potential of spreading COVID rather than stopping it. Furthermore, proper disposal of bio-contaminated everyday mask material is insufficiently regulated even in western countries.

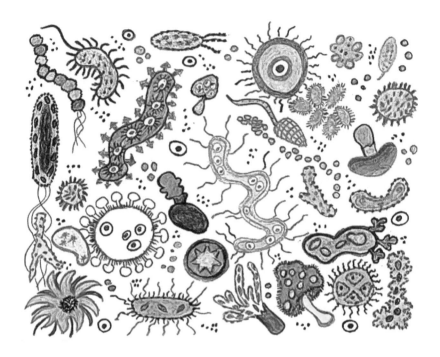

In fact, one of the areas where the environmental impacts of COVID-19 are most pronounced is in waste management. This is a major environmental concern because of the surge in the demand for and the use of plastic products, protective gear, personal protective equipment (PPE), disposable life support equipment and general plastic supplies like syringes, all used in the prevention and treatment of the virus. People are mostly in violation of rules when it comes to disposing of used masks. It has now become common to see used masks scattered everywhere - on sidewalks, public gardens, beaches and in parking areas.

The poor and inadequate waste management strategies within developing and least developed countries contribute to a higher threat of community spread of COVID-19. Public health experts say that improperly discarded masks could be potential sources of the virus if people come into contact with them as the virus can survive on a surgical mask for seven days.

In big cities where thousands of individuals, including children, make their lives working in the streets, coming into contact with these contaminated face masks becomes a constant threat. There is also a high chance for masks to get washed away and end up in oceans, rivers and lakes, affecting flora and fauna negatively. Improper disposal of biomedical waste is responsible for soil and groundwater pollution and adversely affects the biota.

If masks are not discarded properly, they may linger in the environment for up to 450 years and cause huge problems to the environment and our future generations.

Over the medium to long term, animals and plants are affected. Plastic waste can smother environments and break up ecosystems.

Some animals are unable to differentiate between trash and food and end up ingesting the masks. These animals often choke on them and die. Even if they do not choke, animals can become malnourished as the materials fill up their stomachs but provide no nutrients. Smaller animals get entangled in the elastic within the mask as they begin to break apart.

Waterlogged masks, gloves, hand sanitised bottles and other coronavirus waste are already being found on our sea beds and washed up on our beaches.

Already, some 8 million tonnes of plastics enter our ocean every year, adding to the estimated 150 million tonnes already circulating in marine environments.

One study estimates that in the UK alone, if every person used a single-use face mask a day for a year, it would create an additional 66,000 tonnes of contaminated waste and 57,000 tonnes of plastic packaging.

Plastics also break down into smaller pieces over time, and the longer litter stays in the environment, the more it will decompose. Plastics first break down into microplastics and eventually into even smaller nano plastics. These tiny particles and fibres are often long-lived polymers that can accumulate in food chains. Just one mask can produce millions of particles, each with the potential to also carry chemicals and bacteria up the food chain and potentially into humans thereby threatening the entire ecosystem.

Microplastic pollution has contaminated the entire planet, from the summit of Mount Everest to the deepest oceans. People consume tiny microplastic particles via food and water as well as breathing them in. Apparently, people eat at least 50,000 plastic particles a year and breathe in a similar quantity.

Researchers analysed 17 previous studies which looked at the toxicological impacts of microplastics on human cell lines. The scientists compared the level of microplastics and which damage was caused to the cells with the levels consumed by people through contaminated drinking water, seafood and table salt.

The harm included cell death and allergic reactions and the research is the first to show that this happens at levels relevant to human beings. However, the health impact to the human body is uncertain because it is not known how long microplastics remain in the body before being excreted.

Evangelos Danopoulos, of Hull York Medical School who led the research published in the "Journal of Hazardous Materials", said the next step for researchers was to look at studies of microplastic harm in laboratory animals considering that experiments on human subjects would not be ethical. In March 2021, a study showed tiny plastic particles in the lungs of pregnant rats that passed rapidly into the hearts, brains and other organs of their foetuses.

In December 2021, microplastics were revealed in the placentas of unborn babies, which the researchers said was "a matter of great concern". In October 2022, scientists showed that babies fed formula milk in plastic bottles were swallowing millions of particles a day.

Microplastic pollution has also been detected in human blood for the first time, with scientists finding the tiny particles in almost 80% of the people tested.

The findings showed that the particles can travel around the body and may lodge in organs. The impact on health is as yet unknown. But researchers are concerned that microplastic may cause millions of early deaths a year.

The scientists analysed blood samples from 22 anonymous donors, all healthy adults and found plastic particles in 17. Half the samples contained PET plastic, which is commonly used in bottled drinks, while a third contained polystyrene, used for packaging food and other products. A quarter of the blood samples contained polyethylene, from which plastic carrier bags are made. Surgical masks are made of a combination of these types of plastic.

The research is published in the journal "Environment International" and adapted existing techniques to detect and analyse particles as small as 0.0007mm. Some of the blood samples contained two or three types of plastic.

"The big question is what is happening in our body?" Vethaak, one of the researchers, said. "Are the particles retained in the body? Are they transported to certain organs, such as getting past the blood-brain barrier?" And are these levels sufficiently high to trigger disease? We urgently need to fund further research so we can find out."

A recent study found that microplastics can latch on to the outer membranes of red blood cells and may limit their ability to transport oxygen. The particles have also been found in the placentas of pregnant women which could cause the same damaging effects mentioned above in the case of pregnant rats and their foetuses.

A new review paper, co-authored by Vethaak, assessed cancer risk and concluded: "More detailed research on how micro- and nano-plastics affect the structures and processes of the human body, and whether and how they can transform cells and induce carcinogenesis, is urgently needed, particularly in light of the exponential increase in plastic production. The problem is becoming more urgent with each day."

Microplastic fibres were also found deep in the lower lungs of living human beings in almost every person sampled in a recent UK study.

The study from Great Britain discovered microplastic particles in the lung tissue of 11 out of 13 patients undergoing surgery.

Polypropylene (PP) and polyethylene terephthalate (PET) were the most prevalent substances present in the lungs.

The microscopic plastic fragments and fibres were discovered by scientists at Hull York Medical School in the UK. In patients undergoing surgery, some of the filaments found in the sampled lung tissues were two millimetres long.

The plastic dust and microscopic debris comprises the same plastics used to manufacture surgical masks.

Microplastics were detected in human blood for the first time in March, showing the particles can travel around the human body and may become embedded in organs. The impact on health is still to be determined.

Researchers are concerned because microplastics cause damage to human cells in the laboratory and air pollution particles are already known to enter the body and cause millions of premature deaths each year.

"We did not expect to find the highest number of particles in the lower regions of the lungs, or particles of the sizes we found," said Laura Sadofsky, at Hull York Medical School in the UK, a senior author of the study. "It is surprising as the airways are smaller in the lower parts of the lungs and we would have expected particles of these sizes to be filtered out or trapped before getting this deep."

"This data provides an important advance in the field of air pollution, microplastics, and human health," she said.

An older study published in 2020 looked into the risks associated with mask-wearing and the inhalation of microplastics. The study concluded that wearing masks poses microplastic inhalation risk and re-using masks increases the risk.

Chris Schaefer a respirator specialist and expert based in Edmonton has been teaching and conducting respirator fit testing for more than 20 years with his company, SafeCom Training Services Inc.

Schaefer was emphatic when asked if he believed the surgical masks in general use were shedding inhaled microplastics.

"Absolutely. Take a pair of scissors and cut one open. You can see that in between the two main covers that are encapsulating, these loose fibres are breaking away. They're becoming dislodged from the cover itself, just through normal wear and tear and the agitation of putting it on and taking it off," Schaefer said.

"The heat and moisture that it captures will cause the degradation of those fibres to break down smaller. Absolutely, people are inhaling microplastic particles. I've written very extensively on the hazards of these breathing barriers for the last two years, I've spoken to scientists and other people about people inhaling the fibres. If you get the sensation that you've gotten a little bit of cat hair, or any type of irritation in the back of your throat after wearing them," said Schaefer. "That means you're inhaling the fibres."

Schaefer said we will have to wait to see the long-term effects of the inhalation of microplastics from masks.

"So we know that people are inhaling the fibres. What the risks are going to be, what the effects are going to be — it could be anything — but it could definitely cause lung inflammation and could cause full-body inflammation. Absolutely," Schaefer said.

The mask market is also a very profitable venture: the UN trade body, UNCTAD, estimates that global sales totalled around $166 billion in 2020 compared to 800 million dollars in 2019.

Recent media reports are showing videos and photos of divers picking up masks and gloves, littering the waters around about any coastline. This was a wake-up call for many and a reminder that politicians, leaders and individuals need to address this pollution problem.

If historical data is a reliable indicator, it can be expected that around 75% of the used masks, as well as other pandemic-related waste, will end up in landfills, or floating in the seas. Aside from the environmental damage, the financial cost, in areas such as tourism and fisheries, is estimated by the UN Environment Programme (UNEP) at around $40 billion.

The UN Environment Programme (UNEP) has warned that, if the large increase in medical waste, much of it made from environmentally harmful single-use plastics, is not managed soundly, uncontrolled dumping could result.

The potential consequences, says UNEP, which has produced a series of factsheets on the subject, include the already mentioned public health risks from infected used masks, and the open burning or uncontrolled incineration of masks, leading to the release of toxins in the environment, and to secondary transmission of diseases to humans.

Because of fears of these potential secondary impacts on health and the environment, UNEP is urging governments to treat the management of waste, including medical and hazardous waste, as an essential public service. The agency argues that the safe handling, and final disposal of this waste is a vital element in an effective emergency response.

"Plastic pollution was already one of the greatest threats to our planet before the coronavirus outbreak," says Pamela Coke-Hamilton, UNCTAD's director, "The sudden boom in the daily use of certain products to keep people safe and stop the disease is making things much worse."

One February beach clean in Hong Kong found 70 masks along 100 metres of shoreline, with 30 more appearing a week later. In the Mediterranean, masks have reportedly been seen floating like jellyfish. Littered areas also tend to encourage further littering, making the problem worse.

Even the community mask poses an environmental threat, the University College London team examined the manufacture, use and disposal of masks that were disposable, reusable, and reusable with disposable filters, to calculate their overall environmental impact. Perhaps surprisingly, the working paper estimates that hand washing reusable masks with disposable filters had the highest environmental impact overall – even higher than using fully disposable masks.

In conclusion, the whole matter is an utter disaster from whichever perspective we wish to look at it.

My point of view is that the lack of awareness of the planet's homeostatic potential led to the CO_2 hysteria which became the Global Warming, a now proven false theory considering that in the past 15 years the world temperature rose at a normal 0.5° C per century to compensate for the "little Ice age" of mediaeval times. Global warming had, consequently, to be turned into the Climate Change panic which led to the Great Reset.

On this subject a group of over 31000 scientists wrote a petition to the USA government and published a detailed article that gives plenty of data in contrast with the official version on global warming, climate change and anthropogenic cause of climate degeneration. As follows a few points discussed in their article.

"Hydrocarbon use and atmospheric CO_2 do not correlate with the observed temperatures. Solar activity correlates quite well. Correlation does not prove causality, but non-correlation proves non-causality. Human hydrocarbon use is not measurably warming the earth. Moreover, there is a robust theoretical and empirical model for solar warming and cooling of the Earth. The experimental data do not prove that solar activity is the only phenomenon responsible for substantial Earth temperature fluctuations, but they do show that human hydrocarbon use is not among those phenomena.

Temperature rose for a century before significant hydrocarbon use.

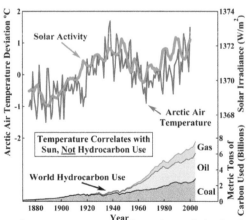

Temperature rose between 1910 and 1940, while hydrocarbon use was almost unchanged. Temperature then fell between 1940 and 1972, while

hydrocarbon use rose by 330%. Also, the 150 to 200-year slopes of the sea level and glacier trends were unchanged by the very large increase in hydrocarbon use after 1940.

Both the sea level and glacier trends – and the temperature trend that they reflect – are unrelated to hydrocarbon use. A further doubling of world hydrocarbon use would not change these trends.

Solar irradiance correlates with them. Hydrocarbon use does not.

This observed variation in solar activity is typical of stars close in size and age to the sun. The current warming trends on Mars, Jupiter, Neptune, Neptune's moon Triton, and Pluto may result from similar relations to the sun and its activity – like those that are warming the Earth.

The Earth has been warming as it recovers from the Little Ice Age at an average rate of about 0.5 °C per century. Fluctuations within this temperature trend include periods of more rapid increase and also periods of temperature decrease.

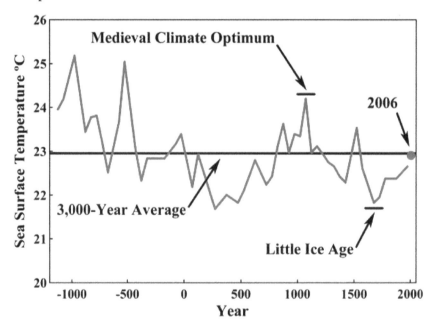

These fluctuations correlate well with concomitant fluctuations in the activity of the sun. Neither the trends nor the fluctuations within the trends correlate with hydrocarbon use. Sea level and glacier length reveal three intermediate uptrends and two downtrends since 1800, as does solar activity. These trends are climatically benign and result from natural processes.

Human production of 8 Gt C (Gigaton of Carbon) per year of CO_2 is negligible as compared with the 40,000 Gt C residing in the oceans and biosphere.

The computer climate models upon which "human-caused global warming" is based have substantial uncertainties and are markedly unreliable.

For example, water vapour is the largest contributor to the overall greenhouse effect. It is a strong greenhouse gas.

On the contrary, the global warming hypothesis with respect to CO_2 is not based upon the radiative properties of CO_2 itself, which is a very weak greenhouse gas.

Methane is also a minor greenhouse gas. World CH_4 (methane) levels are levelling off. In the US in 2005, 42% of human-produced methane was from hydrocarbon energy production, 28% from waste management, and 30% from agriculture.

The "human-caused global warming" – often called the "global warming" – hypothesis depends entirely upon computer model-generated scenarios of the future. There are no empirical records that verify either these models or their flawed predictions.

There is no experimental data to support the hypothesis that increases in human hydrocarbon use or in atmospheric carbon dioxide and other greenhouse gases are causing or can be expected to cause unfavourable changes in global temperatures, weather, or landscape. There is no reason to limit human production of CO_2, CH_4, and other minor greenhouse gases as has been proposed.

We also need not worry about environmental calamities even if the current natural warming trend continues. The Earth has been much warmer during the past 3,000 years without catastrophic effects. Warmer weather extends growing seasons and generally improves the habitability of colder regions.

As coal, oil, and natural gas are used to feed and lift from poverty vast numbers of people across the globe, more CO_2 will be released into the atmosphere. This will help to maintain and improve the health, longevity, prosperity, and productivity of all people.

The United States and other countries need to produce more energy, not less.

Human use of coal, oil, and natural gas has not harmfully warmed the Earth, and the extrapolation of current trends shows that it will not do so in the foreseeable future. The CO_2 produced does, however, accelerate the growth rates of plants and also permits plants to grow in drier regions. Animal life, which depends upon plants, also flourishes, and the diversity of plant and animal life is increased.

Human activities are producing part of the rise in CO_2 in the atmosphere. Mankind is moving the carbon contained in coal, oil, and natural gas from below ground to the atmosphere, where it is available for conversion into living things. We are living in an increasingly lush environment of plants and animals as a result of this CO_2 increase. Our children will therefore enjoy an Earth with far more plant and animal life than that with which we now are blessed."

Another scientist, Piers Corbyn part of the Scientists for truth association share similar scientific views with the above statements and on the CO_2 issues states the following:

"The CO_2 "Climate-Emergency" story says that the trace gas CO_2 (0.04% of air) is the main "control knob" of weather extremes and climate, and that Man's CO_2 – 4% of 0.04% of the atmosphere – is a major dangerous factor in this. Therefore, the story concludes, you must be taxed and controlled. To put that in perspective, imagine if the whole atmosphere is represented by a rod the height of Big Ben's tower (316ft); the level of CO_2 in the atmosphere is about 1.5 inches (38mm) on top and Man's contribution to that CO_2 is between 1 & 2 mm – a pigeon dropping – on top. Look at any Big Ben picture and think about what climate alarmists are claiming!"

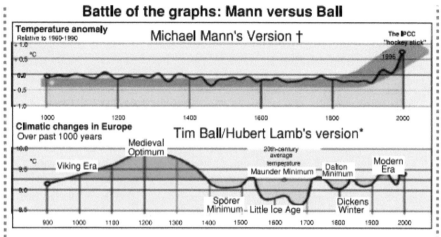

Battle of the graphs: Mann versus Ball

*Originally established by Prof Hubert Lamb (UEA-CRU) and accepted by the IPCC in 1990.
†Hockey stick graph REF.6

Global warmist Iconic Hockey stick graph is fraud - Official

- The contentious - widely shown by the BBC, Exinction Rebelion and the IPCC - "Hockey Stick" graph, showing pretty uniform world temperatures for a thousand years until a recent supposed man made large increase, is now proven fraud.
- The recent court judgement in Canada in which Michael Mann lost his libel against Tim Ball for refusing to provide evidence that his (in)famous graph wasn't fraud means the main icon and evidence of the Global warmist lobby is destroyed.

He also affirms that: "Over a longer period, ice-core data shows that CO_2 levels, follow world climate temperatures with a delay of about 500-800 years. The current increase in CO_2 levels in the last 100 years is an after effect of the medieval warm period. This took place around 500-800 years ago when the climate was warmer than our current period, despite having fewer people burning fewer fossil fuels, by about one degree worldwide and at least two degrees in parts of temperate zones."

Furthermore, lack of Terrain theory awareness has led to compulsive sticking to the Germ theory frenzy which led to obsession with vaccination and antibiotics which in turn led to over-medicated and over vaccinated populations and an overall degeneration of health. In the meantime, the planet heals itself, just like any living creature with homeostatic potentials.

And here I am talking out of direct and personal experience. For a few years I was running the first European "Living Machine" an ecologically engineered sewage treatment plant designed to treat the waste waters of about 500 people living at the Findhorn Ecovillage in the North of Scotland. The wastewater is running through a series of tanks filled with anaerobic and aerobic bacteria, algae, various microorganisms, plants, snails and fish and once cleansed is used for irrigation. In theory the inhabitants of the village had to comply with some basic rules such as avoiding to dispose chemicals and polluting detergents in the toilets.

Unfortunately, and despite the ecovillage designation, the recommendations were highly disregarded and what I was finding in the routinely blocked water pumps is unmentionable.

Despite the damping of bleach, hair conditioner, sanitary towels, socks and various other paraphernalia, the living machine was thriving and producing luxurious plants and vegetables. Even the delicate fish population in the end of the chain of water purification remained alive and breeding just fine. Every Friday, when I was undertaking the weekly chemical tests I was apprehensive that the Living Machine could be unwell or about to perish but I was proven wrong every single time. Nature was far more powerful than 500 inconsiderate humans.

I also believe that CO_2 is a gas fundamental for the sustainment of life. To claim it is a danger does not consider that the actual level of CO_2 is actually too low for an optimal growth of vegetation (it was measured as 416 parts per million in April 2021). If CO_2 is so bad for the planet why are greenhouse growers install CO_2 generators to double plant growth?

More CO_2, produces more vegetation an creates a cooler planet with more oxygen. CO_2 is not the threat. The threats are the synthetic products, the heavy metals and chemicals being unleashed in the environment by the massive industries which are poisoning people and life in general for profit.

The toxins generated by their industries and the alarming levels of microplastic are the cause for environmental concern because those are the toxins that also spread disease and damage the precious ecosystems on the planet.

CHAPTER NINE

Masks: harm to children

"The trick to life is to just keep breathing." – Johnny Lung

Throughout the previous chapters the damage caused by masks to children both on the physical and emotional levels has been largely discussed. However, it felt essential to reserve a space dedicated to this vulnerable and mistreated category.

We have explored developmental issues, adverse reactions and a higher risk of potential damage caused by CO_2 inhalation compared to the one affecting the adult population.

For example, a German study on a total of 25,930 children, determined that "with an average mask wearing time of 270 minutes per day the impairments caused were reported by 68% of the parents. These included irritability (60%), headache (53%), difficulty concentrating (50%), less happiness (49%), reluctance to go to school/nursery (44%), illness (42%) impaired learning (38%) and drowsiness or fatigue (37%)."

In another study 1,951,905 children (1 to 16 years of age) were examined in Sweden, between March 1 and June 30th 2020. Swedish national guidelines stated that social distancing was encouraged, but wearing face masks was not. No child died with COVID-19.

A study revealed how mean IQ scores of young children born during the pandemic have decreased by as much as 22 points while verbal, motor and cognitive performance have all suffered as a result of lockdown.

A study published in the Royal Society Open Science journal found that lockdowns in the UK caused around 60,000 children to suffer clinical depression.

Figures show that 400,000 British children were referred to mental health specialists last year for issues such as eating disorders and self-harm.

Education experts have asserted that forcing schoolchildren to wear face masks has caused long lasting psychological trauma.

An Ofsted report also warned of serious delays in learning caused by lockdown restrictions. "Children turning two years old will have been surrounded by adults wearing masks for their whole lives and have therefore been unable to see lip movements or mouth shapes as regularly," states the report. Another study out of Germany found that the reading ability of children has plummeted compared to pre-COVID times thanks to lockdown policies that led to the closure of schools.

When it comes to children and according to the "hygiene hypothesis," another problem is caused by extremely clean environments that fail to provide the necessary exposure to germs required to "educate" the immune system so it can learn to launch its defence responses to infectious organisms. In his article "A year of COVID-19 lockdown is putting kids at risk of allergies, asthma and autoimmune disease" Byram W. Bridle, Associate Professor of Viral Immunology at the Department of Pathobiology in the University of Guelph expresses many concerns regarding children in the past two years.

The ability of the immune system to self-regulate relies on interactions with the microbial world, especially via interactions with other people, particularly family members. This allows children's immune systems to learn to differentiate between things that are dangerous and those that are not. In turn, their immune system will become equipped to respond to dangers while preventing potentially harmful responses to things that pose no threat, such as inert environmental molecules and normal gut-resident bacteria.

Isolating a young child from non-dangerous microbes in their environment compromises the 'immunoregulatory' components of their immune system. And as explained in the article, a dysregulated immune system often manifests itself in the form of allergies, asthma, and autoimmune diseases.

The core idea he bases his hypothesis on is that "we live in a microbial world: an environment full of bacteria, parasites, viruses and fungi. And that our interactions with these microbes after birth are extremely important to educate our immune systems to function properly. When we are born, our immune systems are still immature and delicate".

Microbiologist Sally F. Bloomfield further explains that: "The immune system is a learning device, and at birth it resembles a computer with hardware and software but few data. Additional data must be supplied during the first years of life, through contact with micro-organisms from other humans and the natural environment."

Bridle also explains that the immune system has many potent mechanisms for killing pathogens. It needs to be carefully regulated to ensure it can eliminate dangerous microbes from the body without causing excessive harm to our own tissues. The interactions we have with our environment early in life are essential for our immune systems to learn to differentiate between safe and dangerous disease-causing microbes.

Our bodies are covered inside and out with micro-organisms that, under normal circumstances, happily reside with us and promote a healthy immune system. If infants, toddlers and young children are not sufficiently exposed to the microbial world around them, their ability to properly regulate their own immune systems can be compromised.

To return to the computer analogy, the data that gets uploaded into the software are incomplete. This lack of data can cause the immune system to struggle to differentiate between what is truly dangerous and should be eliminated, and what is not dangerous and should not be responded to. In a nutshell, this scenario can cause a wide range of illnesses.

Nowadays, scientists are moving away from using the term "hygiene hypothesis" because it could be misinterpreted as meaning that hygiene is not good for a developing immune system. This is not true, nor should anybody advocate eating mud to gain exposure to microbes. Moderation and targeted hygiene would be best.

Specifically, we need to practise proper hygiene in the context of trying to prevent infectious diseases, but still allow our immune systems to interact with safe and essential microbes. Many middle-income countries have seen an epidemic of allergic diseases over the past several decades. This is, in part, due to increased urbanisation which pushes us to living in "concrete jungles" with reduced exposure to the natural environment.

Societies have also adopted behaviours that limit exposure to microbes.

The overuse of antibiotics exacerbates the problem by non-discriminately eliminating good microbes along with bad ones.

Bloomfield and her team of microbiology researchers came to some important conclusions in their study:

"Evidence suggests a combination of strategies, including … increased social exposure through sport, other outdoor activities, less time spent indoors may help reduce risks of allergic disease. Preventive efforts must focus on early life."

Not only mask wearing but all the measures to allegedly prevent COVID diffusion contradict the recommendations to ensure proper immunological development in children.

Data suggest that SARS-CoV-2 does not represent a greater danger to children than the annual flu. Yet social interactions of children have been severely limited, including removing them from schools. Most of their extracurricular activities have been cancelled and they have been discouraged from leaving their homes. Even the air they breathe is often filtered by masks and there is an excessive and harmful use of hand sanitisers.

Most COVID policies have maximised the potential for children to develop dysregulated immune systems.

The problem would likely be more prevalent in infants than toddlers. Although the human immune system is largely mature by approximately age six, some important components are still developing into adolescence.

An unfortunate long-term legacy of this pandemic is likely to be a section of society that grows up to suffer higher-than-average rates of allergies, asthma and autoimmune diseases. This will hold true for children in all countries that enacted isolation policies.

These kids are at greater risk of developing hypersensitivities and autoimmune diseases than anyone before them. The immune systems of children are not designed to develop in isolation from the microbial world.

Throughout the pandemic children have been used as shields in what is ultimately an adult battle over poorly practiced science. Masking is controversial and, arguably, largely ineffective against preventing the spread of viruses in ways other than via coughing and sneezing.

However, they can pose a reasonable barrier to larger environmental particles (e.g. dust particles, dander, pollen, etc.) and bacteria. Through the excessive use of things like antibacterial hand sanitisers, being locked down in homes and lack of physical interactions, we are now well on our way to having a micro-generation of children who will have been isolated like no other human beings in history. Unfortunately, these children will now be part of an unanticipated experiment on a global scale, one to really assess the validity of the so-called 'hygiene hypothesis'.

Children have been forced to wear masks on buses, in schools and at times, even in their own home by hypochondriac and stressed out parents and relatives, in almost every country on this planet. Most of them have been victims of mainstream media induced paranoia.

I am not going to get into the fine details regarding misleading data about 'cases' that have resulted from misuse of PCR and lateral flow tests. Using improperly calibrated testing has caused chronic overestimation of 'cases' of COVID-19 to a substantial but unknown degree. This drove excessive fear. Excessive fear caused our society to abuse children in the name of 'medical science'.

It is shocking to see how many children are still wearing masks even when outdoors with nobody else around, even when in cars with the windows closed. Having experts asked many parents about this, there seem to be three primary reasons: parents are still frightened that their children are at imminent risk of getting infected and dying from COVID-19. Many unmasked parents still insist that their children wear a mask.

A lot of adults have been badly programmed to view children as asymptomatic super-spreaders that will kill grandma.

Many parents are fine with children not wearing a mask but their child is now psychologically addicted to it; either due to fear of dying or causing someone else to die or it has become a security blanket.

The reality is that children are at extremely low risk of dying from COVID-19. What would be much more beneficial to make the risk even lower would be to promote exercise, a healthy diet and bodyweight, time spent outside and sunshine to promote natural production of vitamin D, which the immune system needs for optimal functioning.

Masking children also harms speech development. Observing lip, mouth and tongue placement and movements is critical to the proper development of speech. For example, opposite is a chart known as a 'vowel ladder' used to work with children to improve their pronunciation.

But, masked people is all children have been seeing outside of their home for most of the past 2.5 years, including at school.

A lot of child development specialists are complaining that there has been an increase in speech problems in young children.

For children who know what they want to say but have trouble with pronunciation, adding the muffling effect of a mask makes it even more difficult for others to understand them, so there is a multiplied issue that can cause a lot of frustration.

Vowel Ladder

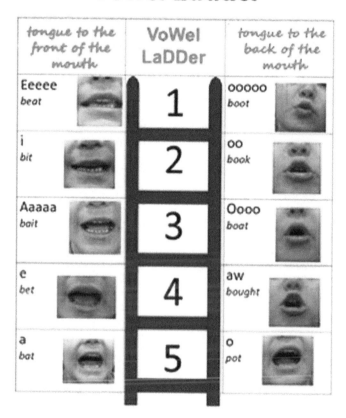

tongue to the front of the mouth	VoWel LaDDer	tongue to the back of the mouth
Eeeee / beat	1	ooooo / boot
i / bit	2	oo / book
Aaaaa / bait	3	Oooo / boat
e / bet	4	aw / bought
a / bat	5	o / pot

I believe that the moral of this story is to stop isolating children from their microbial world. Let them get dirty. Let them interact with other children. Let them hug family members and friends. Consider getting a pet that they can interact closely with. Take them on walks on the beach, in the woods and countryside. Definitely have them wash their hands with soap, but cut down on the antibacterial products and sanitisers. Every time normal flora on the skin is killed, the risks is to re-populated it with pathogens.

Let children see the mouths of others so they can learn to speak properly.

What harm is done from the last two and a half years is done. But, let's not keep locking down, physically distancing and masking children ad nauseam. Not for SARS-CoV-2, not for the annual flu, not for monkeypox, not for anything else, unless it is demonstrated via transparent, objective, publicly disclosed and openly debated science to be a genuine threat to the lives of a substantial proportion of children.

CHAPTER TEN

Masks and dementia care

"For breath is life, so if you breathe well you will live long on earth." —
Sanskrit Proverb

This chapter is mostly based on the findings of a perspective article (and related research) on Frontiers: *Face Masks Protect From Infection but May Impair Social Cognition in Older Adults and People With Dementia* and the Kisielinski et al. German study.

The pandemic has had a huge impact on older adults and people with Alzheimer's disease and other cognitive affected disorders. Masks partially cover the face and debilitate emotion recognition and probably the anticipation of people's intention and their next planned actions. As social cognition is already affected by ageing and dementia, strategies must be developed to cope with these profound changes in communication.

Face masking could even accelerate cognitive decline in the long run. Some studies address face masks' impact on cognition in ageing and dementia, for instance by longitudinally investigating decline before and during the pandemic, and aim to design compensatory strategies. These issues are also relevant for face masking in general, such as in medical surroundings and beyond the COVID-19 pandemic as we have already determined in the previous chapters.

According to Baron, Cohen and other authors' Theory of mind or mind-reading: "social cognition requires, beside others, the understanding of another individual's feelings, intentions, desires and mental states."

Successful social cognition is even more important during extraordinary situations such as the coronavirus pandemic that has become a devastating sanitary and global emergency. In particular, handling such a situation needs optimal communication to understand the event and related measures, and close cooperation between people. The impact of face masking on social cognition and emotion recognition in older adults and people with dementia has had huge effects on the short and long-term.

In the short-term, elderly perform less efficiently in emotion recognition and mind reading, compared to younger adults. This issue is enhanced by mask wearing and certain cohorts are specifically affected, for example individuals with hearing impairment.

This obviously worsens their interaction with partners, caregivers and relatives. In the long-term mask wearing contributes to social isolation, worsening of depression and anxiety, acceleration of cognitive decline and behavioural impairments, development of Subjective Cognitive Impairment (SCI) and Mild Cognitive Impairment (MCI), earlier conversion to dementia, hallucinations, delusion, visual-spatial and executive deficits, unawareness, Developmental Prosopagnosia (DP which is face recognition deficits in the absence of brain damage), delayed recognition and initiation of prevention strategies and therapies.

Those issues are even more prominent in Alzheimer's Dementia (AD), Behavioural Variant Frontotemporal Dementia (BVFTD), Lewy Body Dementia (LBD), Mild Cognitive Impairment (MCI), Posterior Cortical Atrophy (PCA), Primary Progressive Aphasia (PPA), Subjective Cognitive Impairment (SCI), Small Vessel Disease (SVD) and Semantic Variant Primary Progressive Aphasia (SVPPA).

Impact of Face Masking on Social Cognition and aging

As previously discussed masks shield the mouth and the nose and hide about 60-70% of the face area relevant for emotional expression. The mouth region is of particular importance for emotion recognition.

A study by Carbon determines that face masks severely impairs the assessment of the emotional state of another individual and the confidence in one's own assessment ability. Effects appear to be emotion-specific, in accordance with previous studies, showing that the recognition of happiness and sadness, and to a smaller degree anger, rely strongly on the lower part of the face, in particular the mouth. Recognition of disgust is also severely impaired by face masking. Only neutral and fearful faces could be detected in spite of masking, where for fear the eye region provides generally most relevant information for correct recognition. Ageing might even boost this masking effect as older adults have more difficulty in recognising some basic emotions such as disgust, happiness, and fear, and also problems in recognising other basic emotions such as anger and sadness. A limitation of this study, is that relies on visual static stimuli only and disregards recognition of individuals in movement and in different settings.

The "Reading the Mind in the Eyes" Test designed by Baron, Cohen and other authors seems to be a good proxy to investigate social cognition abilities based on the eye region as it investigates mind-reading ability from gaze. This test shows photographs of the eye-region of a person, where the term most appropriately describing the pictured mental state will need to be selected. It is focused mainly on "affective" theory of mind, which enables understanding of others' emotions, affective states, or feelings. The mind-reading ability from gaze was assessed with this test in a very large population-based cohort including 1,603 persons aged between 19 and 79 years.

The study revealed a linear relation between individual test performance scores and age for women and men. Performance declined with ageing in both, women and men, indicating an age-related decline in mind-reading ability from the eyes. The decline in performance was large in women and medium sized in men. A linear regression model confirmed that test performance declined with ageing and showed an association with lower verbal intelligence but not gender.

One might criticise that the "Reading the Mind in the Eyes" test has limitations because it investigates a very specific and rather artificial situation, mind-reading only from the eyes, as in real life other information to judge mental state will be available from context, body language, gestures, language, and non-verbal information. At the same time the study offers a very important insight into this phenomenon.

A study by Chaby et al. investigated gaze strategies accompanying facial emotional processing with ageing. During looking at basic facial expressions, gaze movements were recorded. Older adults performed worse than younger adults in identifying facial expressions, except for joy and disgust. Remarkably, older adults used a focused-gaze strategy as they focused their attention only on the lower part of the face.

On the contrary, younger adults used an exploratory-gaze strategy, repeatedly visiting the upper and lower facial areas. This finding is consistent with the results of a meta-analysis showing that older adults display a bias to look more at the mouth and less at the eyes in facial emotion processing compared to younger adults.

Consequently, older people might lack experience in exploring upper face regions, which is necessary when the lower face is covered by a mask.

Beside emotion recognition, as shown at least for static facial emotions, other abilities for social cognition might be affected. With face masking, people may rely on information from the eyes to attribute mental states to others and successfully interact with them but more analysis is required to fully understand this phenomenon.

A meta-analysis has confirmed the effects of age on social cognition for both, "affective" and "cognitive" theory of mind, where the latter enables understanding of cognitive states, beliefs, thoughts, or intentions. This comprehensive meta-analysis involved 1,462 participants and several types of theory of mind tasks, for example weighing mental states from the eyes, judging stories where a character's behaviour can be best understood by theorising an underlying mental state, identification of emotions and cognitive states from video clips, understanding protagonist's false belief, and recognising social gaffes.

Overall, older adults performed more poorly than younger adults in these tests of theory of mind with moderate effect size for assessing mental states from the eyes.

Another meta-analysis by Ruffman et al. with 1,667 subjects has shown a general age-related decline in emotion recognition in faces, voices, bodies/contexts.

Hayes et al. confirmed this finding in another more recent and more comprehensive meta-analysis on facial emotion recognition in 10,526 older and young adult samples.

Social Cognition in Dementia

Pronounced impairments in social cognition have been reported in neurodegenerative dementia syndromes, recently referred to as neurocognitive disorders, according to meta-analytical evidence.

In particular Behavioural Variant Frontotemporal Dementia (BVFTD) is characterised by early and severe deficits in social cognition with a strong effect as shown in a meta-analysis across several theory of mind tasks such as "Reading the Mind in the Eyes" Test, Faux pas task, sarcasm and first and second order false belief tasks. Here, the "Reading the Mind in the Eyes" test was one of the most impaired tasks. Also a "Reading the Mind in the Eyes" test predicted behavioural variant in fronto-temporal dementia even better than other tests and indicated early conversion to this disease.

Social cognition as tested with theory of mind tasks is also impaired in the most frequent neurodegenerative syndromes, for example Alzheimer's Dementia, Small Vessel Disease and Vascular dementia. Even Mild Cognitive Impairment, which present with an increased probability of converting to dementia in the long-term, has been reported to be associated with medium impairments in theory of mind and facial emotion recognition.

Consequences of Face Masking in the Short Term

These findings are of particular interest during the COVID-19 outbreak as widespread face masking is recommended for disease prevention. As discussed before older people and persons with dementia are impaired in mind-reading from the eyes and emotion recognition.

Studies by Holmes et al. and Pfefferbaum and North have discussed that the COVID-19 pandemic generally will lead to social isolation, emotional distress, and increase the risk for psychiatric illnesses, such as anxiety, depression, self-harm and suicide.

High-risk populations such as older adults or people with dementia might be particularly affected by isolation and loneliness, also in the light of the "digital divide."

Recently, Mok et al. paid particular attention to the profound impact of the COVID-19 pandemic upon older people with Alzheimer's disease and other cognitive disorders. At present, no study has been investigating the specific impact generated potentially by face masking in ageing and dementia beside the one undertaken by Carbon.

Face Masking Affects Social Behaviour

We have determined that face masking impairs static facial emotion recognition (Carbon), which might be particularly relevant in older adults and persons with dementia already compromised in the socio-cognitive domain.

If face masks are used by older persons, people with dementia and their companions, relatives and caregivers, reading emotions and the mind from faces will generally be impeded. Older people and persons with dementia cannot rely on facial emotions as they did previously to convey the emotions/intentions of their caregivers nor to express their intentions/emotions in a way that caregivers can usually understand.

Consequently, social interaction between these persons will be hindered. Individuals might feel isolated, misunderstood and develop depressive symptoms. Face masking is not the only factor that adds to social isolation. There is a need to also consider the other implemented measures such as lock-downs and social distancing.

Impairments of emotion processing and social cognition might not be recognised by relatives and caregivers in older persons due to face masking. Deficits in social communication might further debilitate diagnostic workflows and initiation of appropriate treatment. Subjective and mild cognitive impairment that might increase the risk of being converted to dementia in the long-term might not be early recognised. Accordingly, preventive strategies in cognitively impaired and older people cannot be initiated. This involves but is not limited to physical and mental activity, dietary changes and other indicated therapies. Moreover, symptoms of depression and anxiety increased by these alterations and potentially unrecognised due to face masking, might accelerate cognitive decline.

On one hand, this issue is relevant for every older subject. As discussed before, ageing generally impairs social cognition for both "affective" and "cognitive" theory of mind and emotion recognition.

On the other hand, specific cohorts need special attention. Older adults with hearing loss, a frequent issue in ageing, are prone to problems in social conversation as they cannot anymore rely on their lip-reading skills. This fact is even more important as research has shown an independent association between age-related hearing loss and dementia. The same issue applies for individuals in which English is not the first language.

Comparable problems might appear in persons suffering from communication problems per se, in particular in neurodegenerative primary progressive aphasia.

People with a liability to hallucinations/delusions or severe visual-spatial deficits and prosopagnosia might be unable to recognise persons with face masks correctly, which might be a problem in Lewy body disease, BVFTD,Alzheimer's, posterior cortical atrophy and semantic variant primary progressive aphasia.

Behavioural disease-related impairments might be worsened due to communicative misunderstandings.

Further neuropsychiatric diseases need special attention as social cognitive deficits are already specific symptoms of the disease, for example in Behavioural Variant Frontotemporal Dementia. Based on these arguments one might assume that face masking will deteriorate social cognition and disease course in persons with neurodegenerative disease/dementia, which has to be proven further in future studies.

Finally, effects of face masking on social behaviour might interact with intelligence and gender where higher intelligence/education, and presumably female sex are expected to strengthen coping strategies.

People with combined executive deficits and unawareness, particularly in Behavioural Variant Frontotemporal Dementia, are unable to even recognise the requirement for face masking and, consequently, are unable of using compensatory strategies.

Furthermore, Lara et al. have shown in a meta-analysis that loneliness is associated with Mild Cognitive Impairment and Dementia.

As a consequence, older people, in particular persons with subjective and Mild Cognitive Impairment and in states of risk of dementia, might experience cognitive decline.

Moreover, delayed or even missed diagnosis of cognitive decline due to deficits in socio emotional communication, as discussed before, might hamper recognition and treatment of dementia. Socio emotional communicative deficits add to the generally reduced utilisation of health care services such as day clinics and relief services, visiting general practitioners or taking prescribed therapies as observed in cognitively impaired older persons for instance in Germany during the COVID-19 pandemic. Accordingly, an accelerated cognitive decline could be expected in older people and cognitively impaired during the COVID-19 pandemic. Moreover, more frequent depression might further accelerate this process.

Surprisingly, interpersonal distance was significantly reduced when characters were wearing a face mask compared to characters displaying neutral, happy or angry facial expressions. Interpersonal distance was diminished in participants infected with SARS-CoV-2 or living in low-risk areas. This study contradicts the initial hypothesis that face masking simply increases the awareness for other prevention measures. It underlines the complex consequences of face masking on emotional and social cognition. Study results by Cartaud et al. state that people are more prone to social distancing when characters are not wearing masks, which seems an expected result of face masking.

During the pandemic I have been working in several wards and cared for elderly with mental health issues and a wide range of cognitive disorders. I have experienced the confusion and distress of my patients due to the deprivation of family visits and far too many other restrictions.

I personally believe that it is cruel, inconsiderate, unprofessional and unethical to wear a mask when caring for such vulnerable adults as it in the case of children. It is even worse to force them to comply with the same unscientific and devastating policies.

CHAPTER ELEVEN

Masks and cases

"In individuals, insanity is rare; but in groups, parties, nations and epochs, it is the rule." - Friedrich Nietzsche

This chapter needs no words. Just a brief introduction: a survey conducted by over a dozen medical institutions for the CDC and published in September 2020 showed that 85% of those who contracted COVID-19 during July among the study group either "always" or "often" wore face coverings within the 14 days before they were infected. More than 70% of those outpatient individuals who tested positive reported always wearing masks. Just 3.9% reported never wearing a mask. Here is some further evidence from pictures (source: Our World in data).

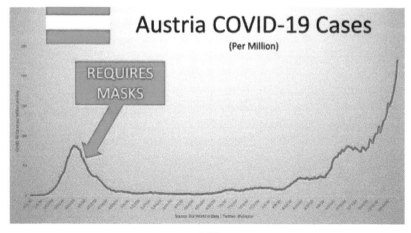

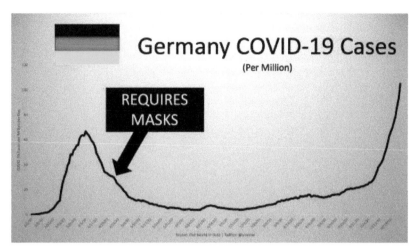

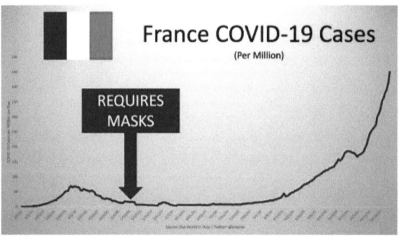

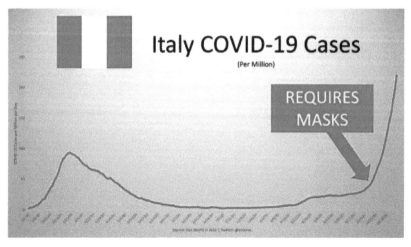

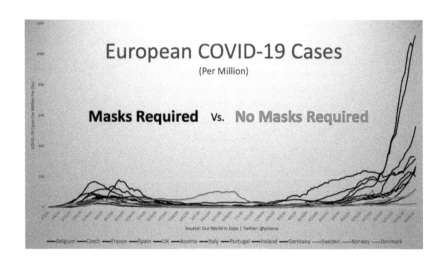

CHAPTER TWELVE

Mass formation, hypochondria and hysteria

"Feelings come and go like clouds in a windy sky. Conscious breathing is my anchor." – Thich Nhat Hanh

In May 2020, our ward clerk posted on social media a BBC article condemning people for going on the beach during a bank holiday. Despite this being perfectly legal and endorsed by the Prime Minister. The picture on the article was recycled from a previous year and did not even represent the reality of the moment. The ward Clerk took this event as an excuse to hold a hate speech platform on social media in which colleagues from various wards had the chance to express their hatred.

The person in question started this, whining about the fact that it had not been possible for her to see her daughter during the first months of the pandemic. Incidentally, I could not see my daughters at home, but bizarrely enough, I could see them at work. Hence, we were booking many shifts in the same locations and we even spent Christmas 2020 in the same ward. The alternative would have been to leave that ward with virtually no staff to cover the shift.

To say that the situation was bizarre is obviously a huge understatement and does not cover the fact that we could not go to my dad's funeral in Italy due to lockdown and we had to invent a creative send off on a local beach. I watched the phenomena in horror.

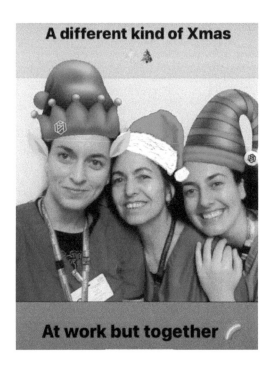

A different kind of Xmas

At work but together

My position at that time was very simple: do you wish to go on the beach within the rules of the law? Go on the beach. Are you scared of beneficial sun rays and to boost your immune system? Do you want to prevent the activation of vitamin D in your body and you still wish to hide in your living room? Please stay at home. Would you like to wear a mask whilst running along the seafront and suffocate yourself to death? Be my guest. Do you want to never come in contact with a face mask? Do not. As long as you leave other people the freedom to do whatever they wish too. Do you want to choose your daughter as the person outside your household that you want to meet? Go and meet your daughter. Do you want to choose another person instead? Do so. But then do not complain that you cannot see your daughter. And especially do not hold hate speech platforms to back you up.

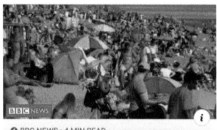

Why Why Why? I desperately want to see my daughter who i haven't seen since 1st February but I'm being sensible and holding off whilst these idiots do this. No common sense or respect for others and the NHS

BBC NEWS

⊕ BBC NEWS · 4 MIN READ
Resort locals 'shocked and angry' at beach crowds

When I saw the shower of nasty comments, at first, I stood in disbelief. My colleagues could not have just said that or anything like it, for that matter. They did though. Not to mention the few "likes" the ward manager put under some of the comments.

It was obvious that if they didn't close the beaches this would happen. I love it that people have the time! People have no common sense. I'd love to go down to the sea but have no intention of doing so as I don't want to get ill.

  ... 1

Unfortunately Boris' speech a few weeks ago had made people think there is less of a risk 🙄
The government need to stop treating the public like they are sensible, and start treating them like idiots!

 💬 ... 1

Why can't the police start fining these twats!

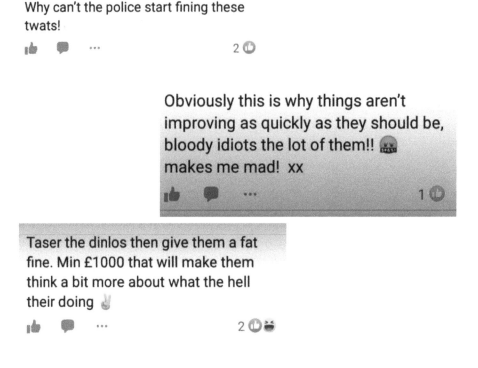

Obviously this is why things aren't improving as quickly as they should be, bloody idiots the lot of them!! makes me mad! xx

Taser the dinlos then give them a fat fine. Min £1000 that will make them think a bit more about what the hell their doing

Stamp their hands with indelible ink. When they get Covid no hospital treatment available due to their irresponsible actions, simple.

I vented my frustration on my own profile:

'Some people I work with, wound up by guess what, a fear mongering BBC article, just posted something asking "why people go on the beach and how irresponsible they are and that they should be fined and if they come to the hospital where we work they should not be treated". I am not going to reply there because I do not want to be hung, stoned to death, or burned at the stake like my ancestor Giordano Bruno. My answer though would be something like: Because to stay indoors/isolation/fear/panic kills you and being in the fresh air/under the sun/socialising and having a good time saves your life? If I could have a guess the "indoor people" will be the second wave and the people having a decent bank holiday will be totally fine."

One of my New York friends replied:

"Those same bigoted medical workers should also say that they will refuse treatment of smokers, because everyone knows smoking is dangerous and very often deadly. Why not also refuse to treat anyone who drives over the speed limit or "jaywalks" across a road and then gets injured? They should refuse to treat anyone who lives in a flood zone or near a volcano or an earthquake zone or near a nuclear facility or chemical plant or military installation, because those people KNOW the danger of living in such a dangerous place, right? Such reckless behaviour must be punished and who better to meet out the punishment than our wonderfully heroic, caring, brave medical workers? Why not be consistent? Be foolish and bigoted on all issues, instead of just about the recent corona panic. Maybe we should ban people from hospitals completely, if we determine that they regularly eat an unhealthy diet or that they do not keep their home clean enough. Should we really allow elderly people into a medical facility, if they are unable to shower regularly? I mean, they might have GERMS on their bodies, which would then endanger the hospital staff. Maybe we should ban infants as well. Infants are the most irresponsible group on earth. Everyone knows how unsanitary their habits are!

Seriously, if they are unwilling to treat any ill or injured people, those medical workers are unfit for their job".

My conclusion on the post was:

"Just to conclude on this post, I am overwhelmed by the love, care, compassion, not to mention the remaining 4C's (courage, communication, commitment, competence) of my colleagues. The way they embody NHS values is astonishingly beautiful. I wish I was one of our patients. Especially one of those marked with indelible ink for being irresponsible".

The irresponsible action being the one of going on the beach with their kids for a couple of hours on a sunny Sunday afternoon. I am proud of being one of such NHS heroes. Especially when those indelible marks remind me of yellow stars, Nazis, concentration camps and related deaths. This is exactly how that one started. For what? I repeat: for a couple of hours with their kids on the beach? If this is not pure insanity I do not know what it is. I am delighted to go back to my ward on Tuesday. NOT."

After long thinking I could not stand back any longer and I wrote this on the ward clerk's profile:

"Each of you works with about 24 colleagues, various "bank" and agency, 18 patients with a high turnover, management, domestics, place of safety and security guards. Double this to consider the two wards. Or even triple that. Many of you also work in several other wards in different hospitals. Again, count the people you get in contact with. Yes, exactly you who are so furious with the people going with kids on the beach for a couple of hours on a sunny afternoon. You and I are touching everything that everyone else touches, spreading infection in different towns and hospitals. We are the ones that should be marked with indelible ink, not them. And the hate speech here is just appalling".

I was trying to point out that, infection control wise, we were far more dangerous than a family going from home to the beach and back.

I was then unfriended and blocked. This came with relief. I was quite bored of the ward clerk daily 'gin and tonic saves you and your family from any ailment' posts. From then on, anytime a patient was verbally approached with a "love" or a "dear", just because the matron was watching, I was having goose bumps.

I sent all of the above to my apprenticeship tutor to ask for her outlook on the matter and a professional and independent opinion. In these days and with all the conflicting views on everything, there was so much confusion and, sometimes, it was no longer easy to determine what was right and what was not.

The tutor, quite alarmed, called me. In the beginning, she had thought that this was a fictional scenario for an essay. But, soon enough, she made an engine search and was able to identify the ward clerk as someone working in my hospital. This shocked her.

In her opinion the ward clerk was in breach of company policies in reference to the use of social media. The clerk's suggestion that she was not able to see her daughter was out of her choice and not a limitation of the law. If she would choose to see her daughter outside her household observing social distancing, this was legally allowed.

Suggesting that people do not respect the NHS because they were going to the beach it was not a valid affirmation and actually did not reflect any NHS' official view. If anything, it gave a wrong impression of the NHS stand on how to deal with individuals simply following legal directives.

Creating a platform that supported radicalised ideas on how to deal with people that actually had done nothing illegal, was dangerous, undermined the NHS and its values and it was ultimately wrong. The public and especially vulnerable individuals with mental health issues, reading the comments on the clerk's platform may have felt intimidated and afraid of contacting the services for fear of having done something wrong and being stigmatised for having visited the beach or the park. They may also have felt that this was the predominant stand within any NHS hospital and jeopardised their health and attendance to appointments. Furthermore, to wind up, radicalise and further values contrary to the ones promoted by the NHS in a group of co-workers was against company policies.

In conclusion the very person that righteously thought that her stand worked in favour of the NHS was the one that actually had no respect for others and the NHS and ultimately undermined the company and its values.

This event had me deeply reflecting on what was going on and the extreme reactions I would observe in people around me and in the general population. This was the first instance and many others followed in the next months such as one of my colleagues frantically and obsessively disinfecting the same door knob for 16 minutes continuously whilst thinking that nobody was watching.

A few days later I saw the following article "The new bigot (popularly called the 'stay-at-home martyr': I am better than you because I enjoy less", written by Riccardo Manzotti in an Italian magazine. Here you can read my translation of the same in English.

"The virus has produced in Italy a new character: the new bigot, popularly called the 'stay-at-home martyr'. In reality what we experience is a form of psychological virus. It's about people that animated by the sacred fury of being right, preach in an obsessive way the respect of anti-infection rules. They pursue this aim and persecute who does not. Like the bigots of past times, these zealous Italians consider themselves as morally superior. For the bigot it is fundamental to trace an insurmountable line between themselves and the rest of the Italians, always described with contempt and indignation. He (or she), obviously, has a sensibility, an understanding of the events, a respect for who suffers, a willingness to sacrifice, that others do not have. He is unlucky, poor soul; he needs to live in a world of people clearly not at his level. Ah! If everybody would just be like him! Unfortunately, he needs to live with the rest of the Country!

The bigot of past times, as the Treccani (most renowned Italian encyclopaedia) teaches us, is a person 'that shows exaggerated zeal more in external practices than in the spirit of the religion, observing with ostentation and pedantry every rule of the cult'. The new bigot is identical: just, instead of religion he has chosen as sacred test the DCPM of the 26th of April on COVID-19. (the equivalent of the COVID 19 act 2020).

The new bigotry, much more contagious than the coronavirus, spreads, like oil stain, in all sectors of the population, even though it has been infecting mostly the lucky ones who can work from home and have less to fear from the economic backlashes of the legislation. But there are exceptions and for that reason nothing can be written in stone.

The new bigot does not open his mouth to criticise the rules, no matter what they are; he just speaks to judge (obviously in a negative way) the other people who do not adapt to the restrictions. And in fact, he makes his voice heard, sometimes from the balconies, with undignified screams, sometimes with warning signs put on the terraces, more often on social media.

Strangely he avoids direct communication. Nearly always, he does not accept dialogue; he seems annoyed by the existence of others and more than everything else by their words. He finds intolerable that someone can put his faith under discussion. Like the old bigot he judges sin severely but even harder who defends it with unsubstantiated argument! The bigot, in fact, trusts just certified sources that he carefully selects on the basis of their conformity with his creed.

A widespread symptom of the new bigotry is the one of banning from their social networks whoever does not share their ideas. In the more acute cases the 'stay-at-home martyr' ceases to answer to calls, emails or text messages from people that are not as pure as him: he fears to be contaminated by the words of whoever is not as faithful as him. Better off to defend his eyes and ears from those shameless shows.

In the beginning bigotry, as all illnesses, manifests itself in three very distinguishable ways: fear, frustration, envy.

To start with, the new bigot is a phobic who experiences news about the virus with great apprehension. Fear pushes him into meticulously adopting every prevention rule. So far, bigotry is asymptomatic and, with luck, it does not develop in its acute form. He stays in a condition of generic apprehension. In many, unfortunately, the combination of fear and limitation of freedom kicks off the acute form!

After a few days of house arrest, the bigot does no longer suffer for the limitations of his freedom, but starts to feel a subtle pleasure: finally, he feels he is in the position of demonstrating his moral superiority over others. This is the first unmistakable symptom that the pathology has started. Where others complain, he endures with patience and diligence. Where others protest, undoubtedly for no edifying reasons, he is silent and obeys. The difference could not be clearer.

At this stage envy and frustration manifest themselves.

Bigotry, as in its traditional form, nourishes itself with the envy that who follows the rules feels for who does not. Clearly, there is an injustice, made even more burning from the fact that who is less virtuous enjoys more.

And this creates frustration.

From his shut window the 'stay-at-home martyr' spies who goes outside, careless of his fear and of his desires of mortification and within himself he feels some envy and frustration that can just find relief in formulating apocalyptic threats: "you will see what is going to happen, they will make us stay at home for ever, the quarantine will become permanent". The bigot does not really manage to enjoy his auto inflicted penance and so wishes in his heart, to whom is not like him, Dante's punishments, end of the world scenarios, a final and no far away judgment day in which the sinners will be at last punished for their lack of morality.

The bigot praises purifying practices, even if useless from a hygienic point of view, such as sanitising the streets; condemns harmless behaviours such as outings or children playing. He does not reason, he judges. He does not think, he believes. He does not wish, he obeys.

Like the flagellants in the middle ages, who in fact are the ones that introduced self- mortification practices, the 'stay-at-home' punishes himself: he wears masks whilst driving, he washes his hands when going between the bedroom and the kitchen, he is planning to stay at home for ever, way beyond the day established by the government, he self-prohibits any contact with friends and family even when the quarantine should have reduced the risk of infection below any critical level, he wears multiple masks (I have seen this many times) even to carry the rubbish to the bins under his flat. These are not hygienic practices; they are spiritual exercises, purification pathways, human sacrifices.

Unfortunately, bigotry once it has reached this stage becomes chronic.

Bigots keep pursuing new measures to limit their own freedom and, just because they do so, they increase their frustration against everybody else, now perceived with augmented annoyance and disdain. If prior the development of the illness they had a generic envy for other people's behaviour, after the acute stage, and having limited themselves, they have become even more envious, in a spiral of growing desire of mortification and aversion for other people's freedom.

The pleas for reason of friends and acquaintances are of no avail, useless to mention percentages and common sense.

The 'stay-at-home martyr' wants to demonstrate that his sacrifice is the only way to safety or, as a second option, that the immorality and thoughtlessness of others will bring disaster.

We have seen this in the days of the reopening in May, when the 'stay-at-home, would rip their clothes forecasting that the Country would end up in the prey of the irresponsibility of everybody.

Instead, nothing happened.

We see this every day when the tiniest sign of joy - like when those young people were dancing in the streets (with masks and social distancing) - gives rise on the lips of the self-righteous to declarations of disdain, requests of repression, moral judgement, proclamations of imminent apocalypse and even invocation for asteroids to bring us to extinction.

The 'stay-at-home martyr' finds comfort in the words of his sacred book, the Giuseppe Conte's gospel, where, at article 1, section G you read: "playful or recreational activity are not allowed; it is only allowed individual sport or physical activity". In these words, the new bigot glimpses the omen that it is his personal sacrifice that will purify us from the virus. In fact, the DCPM condemn spirit but not matter, playful activity but not physical one, dancing but not gym, pleasure but not repetition: movement is allowed but play is not! And why? Considering that the difference between playful and physical is not evident from a health point of view? It is obvious to anyone that the virus does not distinguish a movement done with playfulness or to exercise. It is because play is freedom and joy.

Again, according to the Treccani, in fact, a playful activity is something with "particular reference to the aspect of freedom and joy, mostly separated from rules"

Play, to simplify, is joy and freedom, the very two things that the bigot has decided to eliminate from his life in the name of a presumed moral superiority. Unfortunately, the only efficient vaccine against bigotry:

reason and critical thinking, functions just if inoculated a young age.

In most of the subjects hit at advanced age, bigotry will stay in its chronic form and it will manifest itself every single time it will see joy and freedom."

After reading this article I said to myself: Bingo! Mass psychology can easily explain what is going on in the world nowadays. Consequently, I started to explore the literature and the concept of 'bigotry as mental illness' and the reasons behind hypochondria events throughout the centuries discovering that, as usual, they were very common and standardised phenomena.

In my investigation I explored racism and intolerance towards minorities and how majority 'consensus reality' is reached and the effects that this has on the different, the dissidents and the few.

Eventually, I came across Matias Desmet, a professor of clinical psychology at Ghent University (Belgium) and a psychoanalytic psychotherapist. Desmet is the author of over one hundred peer-reviewed academic papers as well as having a master's degree in statistics. In 2018 he received the Evidence-Based Psychoanalytic Case Study Prize of the Association for Psychoanalytic Psychotherapy, and in 2019 he received the Wim Trijsburg Prize of the Dutch Association of Psychotherapy.

Desmet has been influenced by Hannah Arendt who wrote the famous book "The Origins of Totalitarianism", published in 1951. She was a fugitive from Nazism and had expatriated in America before the Second World War. In her new homeland she studied imperialism, racism and anti-semitism which lead her to conduct the trial on the Nazis war-criminal Adolf Eichmann's in 1961, in Israel. Arendt depicted Eichmann, who helped bring about the Holocaust, as an "unreflective but ambitious bureaucrat essentially unaware of the enormity of his actions in the mass extermination of Jews". Arendt speculated that "Eichmann personified the 'banality of evil'." Although her interpretation was often contested, her description of an ordinary bureaucrat capable of executing monstrosities without conscience never lost its significance since then.

In the most recent book: "The Psychology of Totalitarianism", Desmet gives his interpretation of the past two years from a collective sociological and psychological point of view in the frame of the concepts of mass formation and mass psychosis.

The term 'mass formation' derives from the French author Gustav Le Bon's book "The Crowd: a Study of the Popular Mind", published in 1895. Examples of the mass formation phenomenon can be observed in many past instances: the Medieval witch hunts, the French Revolution, Fascism, Stalinism and Nazism, phenomena that would ruin whole nations and could have even posed a threat to civilisation.

Today, argues Desmet, "We have with the coronavirus crisis…reached a point where the entire world population is in the grip of a mass formation over a prolonged period of time."

Desmet explains that mass formation derives from the manifestation of four psychological conditions at the population level, "feelings of social isolation, the absence of meaning in life, free-floating anxiety (lacking a clear object) and free-floating anger and frustration. Suddenly the lonely, lost and anxious individual can contribute meaningfully to a (allegedly) worthy project. Many thus regain a sense of purpose and feeling of fellowship from doing right by their fellow citizens through the sacrifice of the personal to the (supposed) good of the collective. This is accompanied by intolerance of dissident voices, an informant mentality, susceptibility to pseudo-scientific indoctrination and propaganda, and the blind following of a narrow logic impervious to counter-evidence and transcending ethical boundaries. A new social bond, even a new kind of citizenship, can emerge", says Desmet.

This is the most important aspect of mass formation. It is maintained by persistent messages "injected on a daily basis via mass media, as alternative voices are systematically silenced (especially on masking and distancing) and willingness to receive experimental vaccines – provide a sense of purpose."

"The crowd acts in a coordinated way and repeats the same slogans," Desmet notes. "It engages thoughts and expressions that spread through its ranks at lightning speed. This occurred in Nazi Germany – and during COVID-19."

His main concerns originate from "the increasing government intrusion on individual life, which is growing tremendously fast. Privacy rights are eroding, dissenting voices are being suppressed in multiple areas - especially, in his view, on climate change - and state security forces are acting against their own populations."

Furthermore, with the growing calls for "strict government controls from within the population itself" in Desmet's opinion, all the ingredients are in place for "the emergence of a new totalitarianism, no longer led by flamboyant 'mob leaders' such as Joseph Stalin or Adolf Hitler but by dull bureaucrats and technocrats."

This is why the book's focus is not on "concentration camps, indoctrination or propaganda" but the "totalitarianism that arises from evolutions and tendencies that take place in our day-to day lives."

"Individuals are typically not uniform in their mass formation response", Desmet argues - "about 30% fully internalise the process, become completely committed and willingly promote the narrative. A middle 40-50% is not completely convinced" - but complies to survive the crisis, especially if important aspects of their lives are at risk, such as employment, close relationships or similar and fundamental factors. "The final 10-30% remain independent in their thinking and some engage in outright dissent."

Intelligence and education are no protection against totalitarianism. As an example, nearly half of Germany's medical doctors became Nazi supporters, a much higher percentage than any other profession.

In fact, the highly educated can be the most receptive to mass formation especially when science is constantly cited and used as a manipulative tool.

Desmet raises profound questions about the uses, abuses and limitations of rationality, science and technology and their role in creating a deeply disturbing mass psychological phenomenon. Desmet's analysis shows how whole populations, compelled to operate using a technological mindset that sees science as the answer to everything, can be overtaken by totalitarianism. Desmet believes this was occurring in the pandemic's earliest days and continues today. "This threatens to render science basically just another instrument of politics and their agenda of promotion of products, spreading of deception, furtherance of political programmes and the belittling and stigmatising of those who disagreed."

For example, when Sweden, chose to avoid lockdowns and school closures, outraged academic modelling predicted 80,000 COVID-19 deaths. When the number reached only 6,000, it seemed that the same academics were disappointed and so was the public.

I also noted how the fanatical nature of masking proponents has reached near cult-like levels of obsessive adherence to 'health and safety' dogmas. Inexplicably, after mask mandates were lifted, many were unhappy about it. In fact, countless people are demanding the reinstatement of mandatory mask measures. Is this merely a case of Stockholm Syndrome, or is there something else at play?

Desmet was also among those noticing how the PCR tests, acclaimed as the gold standard, were generating massive numbers of false positives, multiplying the number of reported 'cases'. Public health agencies also began reporting anyone testing positive as a COVID-19 "case" even when affected by other conditions.

For example, under rigorous statistical scrutiny, hospitals in Scotland "were left with 13 percent of the original number of COVID-19 patients."

Desmet actually believes that the very object of totalitarianism is "to pursue pseudo-scientific basis and falsely accepting that a utopian society can be attained from scientific knowledge." Desmet has also extended worries about the failings of scientific research. "For example, in economics research, replication failed about 50 percent of the time, in cancer research about 60 percent of the time, and in biomedical research no less than 85 percent of the time, the quality of research is so atrocious that the world-renowned statistician John Loannidis published in 2005 an article entitled 'Why Most Published Research Findings Are False'."

Desmet is especially worried by the widespread intolerance shown towards dissenting voices. "The way in which unvaccinated people are denied access to parts of public spaces, which even now engenders support within the population for denying them access to grocery stores and hospitals, evokes the most unpleasant reminiscences and may indeed become the first step of an infernal cycle of dehumanisation," he writes.

In conclusion, Desmet believes the most important questions that humanity must ask are not scientific but philosophical, ethical and ideological: "Do we view man as a biochemical machine that has to be technologically monitored and pharmaceutically adjusted, or as a being that finds its destination in mystical resonance with the Other and with the eternal language of nature?" In his mind, the answer is obvious and also offers the path away from totalitarianism.

"Uncertainty and risk will always be with us"- Desmet writes - "but by recognising that uncertainty is inherent in the human condition and by defying the associated anxiety, we can create the conditions for the re-emergence of creativity, individuality and human connectedness and lives based, finally, on ethical and moral choices tried and tested in our communities and civil society. "

On the other hand, totalitarianism, "has its roots in the insidious psychological process... a kind of group hypnosis that destroys ethical awareness robbing people of their ability to think critically."

CHAPTER THIRTEEN

Masks and death

"Look, when you're breathing, you're alive aren't you? Everything is. And when you stop breathing, your heart stops, and then you're dead."

– Susan Hill

A new medical journal report comparing COVID fatality rates across Kansas counties during the pandemic concludes that mask mandates could be associated with higher death rates from the virus.

The observational study *The Föegen Effect: A Mechanism by Which Facemasks Contribute to the COVID-19 Case Fatality Rate* was published in "Medicine" in February 2022 by German doctor Zacharias Föegen.

The paper analysed "whether mandatory mask use influenced the case fatality rate in Kansas" during the time period of August 1st, 2020 to October 15th. Kansas was used for comparison because the state allowed each of its 105 counties to decide whether or not to implement mask mandates, with 81 counties deciding against the measure.

One of the starting points of the research is that in current studies "a lot less focus has been centred on the course of the disease while using masks. This is a questionable approach, as the question "how many lives can be saved?" is more important than the question "how many infections can be prevented?".

Therefore, the aim of the study was "to assess the influence of mask mandates on Case Fatality Rate (CFR) by comparing the CFR between two groups, one with and the other without mask mandates. The corresponding two-sided hypothesis is that mask mandates change the CFR. While an increase in CFR may look unintuitive at first glance, more intuitively, one would not exchange his face mask with another person out of fear to breathe in the virus that is caught in the face mask and get infected. Thus, breathing in one's own virus might increase the CFR".

"The most important finding from this study is that contrary to the accepted thought that fewer people are dying because infection rates are reduced by masks, this was not the case," concluded the paper. "A parallelisation analysis based on county-level data showed that in Kansas, counties with mask mandate had significantly higher case fatality rates than counties without mask mandate, with a risk ratio of 1.85 for COVID-19-related deaths. Even after adjusting for the number of "protected persons," that is, the number of persons who were not infected in the mask-mandated group compared to the no-mask group, the risk ratio remained significantly high at 1.52. By analysing the excess mortality in Kansas, this study determines that over 95% of this effect can solely be attributed to COVID-19. In conclusion: "Results from this study strongly suggest that mask mandates actually caused about 1.5 times the number of deaths or ~50% more deaths compared to no mask mandates."

This means that the risk for the individual wearing the mask should even be higher, because there is an unknown number of people who either do not obey mask mandates, are exempted for medical reasons or do not go to public places where mask mandates are in effect. These people do not have an increased risk and thus the risk on the other people under a mask mandate is actually higher.

The study also gave a potential reason for the disparity in risk ratio (RR) for dying from COVID-19:

"A rationale for the increased RR by mandating masks is probably that virions that enter or those coughed out in droplets are retained in the face mask tissue, and after quick evaporation of the droplets, hyper condensed droplets or pure virions (virions not inside a droplet) are re-inhaled from a very short distance during inspiration."

The theory suggests that COVID-19 "virions spread (because of their smaller size) deeper into the respiratory tract."

"They bypass the bronchi and are inhaled deep into the alveoli, where they can cause pneumonia instead of bronchitis, which would be typical of a virus infection. Furthermore, these virions bypass the multilayer squamous epithelial wall that they cannot pass into 'in vitro' and most likely cannot pass into 'in vivo'. Therefore, the only probable way for the virions to enter the blood vessels is through the alveoli"

"These findings suggest that mask use might pose a yet unknown threat to the user instead of protecting them, making mask mandates a debatable epidemiological intervention," concludes the paper.

In short, the paper's findings are based on the theory of the so-called "Föegen effect," which, as described above, starts from the hypothesis that hyper condensed droplets caught by masks, re-inhaled and introduced deeper into the respiratory tract, could be responsible for the increased mortality rate.

The fundamentals of this effect are easily demonstrated when wearing a face mask and glasses at the same time by pulling the upper edge of the mask over the lower edge of the glasses. Droplets appear on the mask when breathing out and disappear when breathing in. Moreover, the "Föegen effect" could increase the overall viral load because virions that should have been removed from the respiratory tract are returned. Viral reproduction in vivo, including the reproduction of the re-inhaled virions, is exponential compared with the mask-induced linear droplet reduction.

Therefore, the number of exhaled or coughed out virions that pass through the face mask might, at some point, exceed the number of virions shed without face masks. Furthermore, the hyper condensed droplets and pure virions in the mask might be blown outwards during expiration, resulting in aerosol transmission instead of droplet transmission. Moreover, these two effects might be linked to a resurgence of rhinovirus infections.

The use of "better" masks (FFP2, FFP3) with a higher droplet-filtering capacity probably should cause an even stronger "Föegen effect" because the number of virions that are potentially re-inhaled increases in the same way that outward shedding is reduced.

Another salient point is that COVID-19-related long-term effects and multi-system inflammatory syndrome in children may all be a direct cause of the "Föegen effect." Virus entry into the alveoli and blood without being restricted to the upper respiratory tract and bronchi and can cause damage by initiating an auto immune reaction in most organs.

Regarding the proposed consequences of the "Föegen effect, "the question arises, which share of the global death toll and long-term effects of COVID-19 can be attributed to widespread mask use."

The scientific legitimacy of this study was also echoed by Dr Aaron Kheriaty while discussing it during a Saturday night appearance on Fox News' "Unfiltered" with Dan Bongino:

"There is emerging evidence, from a study out of Kansas that recently suggested that the case fatality rate with COVID is higher where there are mask mandates," Kheriaty said. "Once you get infected, if you are wearing a mask, this study suggested that your chance of having a bad outcome, of dying from COVID was higher. And that probably has to do with rebreathing these kinds of condensed droplets that have a lot of virus in them."

While several recent reports, including the University of Louisville study, have shown mask mandates to have had no discernible effect on COVID-19 case rates through the pandemic, the possibility that widespread and prolonged mask usage could actually have negative consequences has largely been ignored by researchers until recently.

In April, a peer-reviewed study comparing mask usage across Europe during the pandemic found that "countries with high levels of mask compliance did not perform better than those with low mask usage," and the analysis also discovered a "moderate positive correlation between mask usage and deaths which suggests that the widespread use of masks at a time when an effective intervention was most needed, for example during the strong 2020-2021 autumn-winter peak, was not able to reduce COVID-19 transmission and that the universal use of masks may have had harmful unintended consequences."

The peer-reviewed study: *Correlation Between Mask Compliance and COVID-19 Outcomes in Europe* was conducted by Beny Spira, an Associate Professor at the University of São Paulo whose research focuses on the molecular genetics of microorganisms.

Published in the Cureus Journal of Medical Science on April 19th, 2022, the paper describes its purpose as "analysing the correlation between mask usage against morbidity and mortality rates in the 2020-2021 winter in Europe".

"Data from 35 European countries on morbidity, mortality, and mask usage during a six-month period were analysed and crossed," and encompassed a total of 602 million people.

"The positive correlation between mask usage and cases was not statistically significant, while the correlation between mask usage and deaths was positive and significant. The Spearman's correlation between masks and deaths was considerably higher in the West than in East European countries."

Spira also explains how confounding factors that could have potentially influenced the study such as vaccination rates or prior levels of COVID-19, were irrelevant: Concerning disparate vaccination rates between countries, he explained "this is unlikely given the fact that at the end of the period analysed in this study (31st March 2021), vaccination rollout was still at its beginning, with only three countries displaying vaccination rates higher than 20%: the UK (48%), Serbia (35%), and Hungary (30%), with all doses counted individually."

"It could also be claimed that the rise in infection levels prompted mask usage resulting in higher levels of masking in countries with already higher transmission rates. While this assertion is certainly true for some countries, several others with high infection rates, such as France, Germany, Italy,

Portugal, and Spain had strict mask mandates in place since the first semester of 2020. In addition, during the six-month period covered by this study, all countries underwent a peak in COVID-19 infections, thus all of them endured similar pressures that might have potentially influenced the level of mask usage," he added.

In support of the 'mask causing death hypothesis' there is also the controversial discussion on the mortality causes and effect of the 1919 "Spanish flu".

A 2008 study co-authored by Dr Anthony Fauci explains that the influenza virus destroyed cells that line the bronchial tubes and lungs which created a pathway for bacteria that normally inhabit the nose and throat to invade the lungs and cause bacterial pneumonia. The study affirms: "The weight of evidence we examined from both historical and modern analyses of the 1918 influenza pandemic favours a scenario in which viral damage followed by bacterial pneumonia led to the vast majority of deaths. In essence, the virus landed the first blow while bacteria delivered the knockout punch."

Of course, the "fact checkers" do the usual perverted and contorted logic exercise in trying to prove that mask wearing did not cause or at least exacerbate the incidence of bacterial pneumonia and consequently the raise in mortality rate. Well, the scientific evidence reported in this chapter and in particular the Föegen effect study just prove them, once more, wrong: mask wearing is a strong contributing factor in bacterial pneumonia and death.

Of course, those with some common sense and the ability to follow scientific data knew that masks are unhealthy from the start of the pandemic. Still, it's psychologically comforting to read that the research is finally catching up.

CHAPTER FOURTEEN

Conclusions

"Inhale, then exhale. That's how you'll get through it."
– Unknown

Having explored the literature and the research there is clear evidence that mask wearing causes adverse effects on all levels: physical, emotional, social, sociological and psychological.

Public health institutions such as the WHO, the European Centre for Disease Prevention and Control (ECDC), the USA Centre for Disease Control and Prevention (CDC) or the German RKI cannot prove with solid scientific data or evidence-based medicine any positive effect of surgical masks in relation to reduced rate of spread of COVID-19 in the population or any decrease in death rates.

In addition, the compulsory wearing of masks gives a deceptive feeling of safety and from an epidemiological point of view, increases the risk of self-contamination and the accumulation of bacteria, fungi and viruses within the masks.

Mask wearers also exhale smaller particles (size 0.3 to 0.5 μm) than mask-less people and this increased fine aerosol production (nebuliser effect) with all the related negative consequences.

Modern history shows that in each and every influenza epidemic (1918–19, 1957–58, 1968, 2002, 2004–2005, 2009) mask impositions could not achieve the hoped for results in the battle against infection.

A plethora of scientific studies do not demonstrate any significant positive effect in mask mandates and various authorities and organisations deem masks as unsuitable to protect the users from viral respiratory infections. Even in hospital use, more and more research on surgical masks point in the direction of the scarce evidence of providing any protection against viruses.

 Mask wearing is also responsible for creating a vicious circle in which its symbolical protection also flags fear of infection followed by collective panic constantly nurtured by the main stream media.

As Neil Oliver rightly explains:

"If the authorities ever genuinely thought that the masks were about health then that was for a very brief period, and I'm not sure they ever did. Ever since that point, it has always and only been about control. It was about muzzling people. Isolating people and splitting people into polarised camps because the last thing that any authoritarian-minded government wants is a confident educated independent population able to make its own decisions and go about its business. Fear has always been the key. There are those for whom the mask is a badge of imagined superiority. There were those who swallowed the hook, line and the sinker that wearing a mask was a good thing to do. Good thing in block capitals. And having shown to be doing the good thing they won't let that drop. Masks make so easy to distinguish the good guys from the bad guys. Masks were always the most straightforward and the most obvious tool to show whether or not people were complying, which team they were on. Which team are you? Team good people who wears masks or team naughty people? It is a really important compliance device."

Furthermore, the recommendation to use masks not out of self-protection but out of "altruism" is another contorted logic by-product of mass mask wearing in many countries in the world.

The ego equates following the rules with being a good virtuous person. We all remember the actor in the adverts stating: "I wear a face covering to protect my mates" Following the rules translates into being a good person, the flip side is, of course, that you are a bad person if you do not.

From a psychological point of view masks are a very important maintainer of fear and we know fear has been artificially elevated throughout the pandemic. Even now masks are acting to keep that fear level going.

When you look around and you detect that other people are wearing masks what does your lizard brain tell you? Hazard, risk, threat, frightening. This amps up people's fear.

Studies show that the major efficacy of a mask is that it causes alarm in the other person.

When you walk down the street and everybody coming towards you has a mask on, you definitely do social distancing. It is just a gut thing.

Many politicians and advisors will admit privately that the policies that compelled people to wear masks were not really about the spread of infection at all but about the psychological effect that they would have. The real purpose is social control to provide a constant reminder to maintain distance from other people, to maintain a state of anxiety that leaves people more likely to comply with the restrictions that might otherwise be resisted or forgotten and this is pretty much exactly what the New Zealand Ministry of Health say in a response to an official freedom of information request from October 2021. This institution says:

"Maintaining the requirement for face coverings provides wider benefits that support the overall response to the pandemic. Face coverings are a constant reminder of the ongoing threat posed by COVID-19 and will help prompt people to be more vigilant about other important behaviours such as physical distancing, using the COVID tracer app, hand hygiene and coughing and sneezing etiquette."

Likewise, in the UK, a report prepared by the SAGE's behavioural science subgroup Spy B was presented for ministerial discussion on the 23rd of march 2020. This document showed that the British government was using applied behavioural psychology inside the COVID science group to make people frightened. The document clearly states as one of the recommendations: "Use the media to increase the sense of personal threat", which translates into: 'use the media to make people fearful'. Now that has not much to do with viral transmission.

The Government planned this intervention on the public, despite the fact that causing an excessive fear in a community does have huge costs, including the tens of thousands of excess deaths that we have seen throughout the pandemic with people, still to this day, being too scared to go into hospital, elderly people dying of loneliness and isolation and the huge increase in suicide rates.

Laura Dodsworth, in her book: "A state of fear" interviewed Kevin Morgan, an educational psychologist who sits on the Spy B behavioural science subgroup of sage. He said: "My day job is running the behavioural insights team known as the 'nudge unit' and we spend a lot of time helping governments across the world using different techniques. The three most prominent psychological nudges that have been deployed on the people of our country are: fear inflation, shaming, and peer pressure or scapegoating."

I don't think it is any coincidence that masks enforce and enhance each of those three nudges in a big way. They are fear perpetuators because it screams at us that one of us is a biohazard or maybe both of us are a biohazard. It also allows people to be identified so that people can tell who is who. Who is following the rules and who is not so it harnesses peer pressure and scapegoating.

But did the mask really help? Did the mask keep the virus out? Almost certainly not. Masks have come to represent a whole range of values and signals.

Recent data suggest that there is no correlation between SARS-CoV-2 reduction in infection rates and mask use. The groups examined show that approximately 70% of the "infection cases" always wore masks and a further 14.4% of them frequently.

From what we explored in the previous chapters, masks appear to be not only less effective than expected, but also liable to cause undesirable biological, chemical, physical and psychological side effects.

Dermatological studies were the first to demonstrate the adverse effects of increases in temperature and humidity that produce, eczema, skin damage, overall impaired skin barrier function and mechanical irritation causing acne in up to 60% of wearers.

From these direct effects many other further detrimental consequences, involving other organs and systems were discovered, especially with regard to the disruptive influence on breathing, respiratory physiology and gas metabolism of the body.

This is particularly important considering that those functions play a key role in maintaining a healthy and sustaining balance in the entire human physiology.

It was determined that the dead space volume is almost doubled by wearing a mask and that a more than doubled breathing resistance leads to the rebreathing of carbon dioxide at every cycle of inhalation and exhalation. A pathological increase in the carbon dioxide partial pressure ($PaCO_2$) in the blood was also observed. This is more worrying in the case of already vulnerable and ill individuals.

According to primary studies, these changes contribute to an increase in respiratory frequency and depth with a corresponding increase in straining of the respiratory muscles. This often causes drops in oxygen saturation (SpO_2) in the blood, already reduced by increased dead space volume and breathing resistance.

The overall drop in oxygen saturation of the blood and the increase in carbon dioxide contribute to an increased stress response, causing heart rate and respiratory rate to rise, in some cases also producing a significant blood pressure increase.

Even minimal changes in blood gases such as those provoked by wearing a mask cause reaction in vital control centres in the central nervous system (locus coeruleus in the brainstem, nucleus solitarius in the medulla) and the activation of the sympathetic axis via chemoreceptors in the carotids.

A link between disturbed breathing and cardiorespiratory diseases such as hypertension, sleep apnoea and metabolic syndrome has been scientifically proven. Decreased oxygen levels together with increased carbon dioxide in the blood stream are considered the main triggers for sympathetic stress response.

Clinical effects of prolonged mask-wearing would consequently cause intensification of chronic stress reactions and negatively influence the metabolism leading to metabolic syndrome.

A connection between hypoxia, sympathetic reactions and leptin release is scientifically known. Leptin is a hormone released by the adipose tissue (body fat). It helps the body maintain your normal weight on a long-term basis. It does this by regulating hunger and providing the sensation of satiety (feeling full). This has obvious implications that may lead to obesity or, on the opposite side of the spectrum, anorexia.

It is also important to consider the connection between breathing and its influence on other bodily functions, including psychological effects and the generation of positive emotions and drive.

The latest findings from neuro-psychobiologircal research indicate that respiration influences brain centres and, consequently helps to shape psychological and other bodily functions and reactions. Since masks impede the wearer's breathing and accelerate it, they work completely against the principles of health-promoting breathing techniques used in holistic medicine and yoga. According to recent research, undisturbed breathing is essential for happiness and health and masks work, once more, against this.

Significant changes in blood gases causing hypoxia (drop in oxygen saturation) and hypercapnia (increase in carbon dioxide concentration) through masks has the potential to have a clinically relevant influence on the human organism such as psychological and physiological reactions on a macroscopic and microscopic level, alteration of gene expression and metabolism on a molecular cellular level, even without exceeding normal limits.

At the cellular level, for example it is important to mention the activation of the hypoxia-induced factor (HIF). HIF regulates cellular oxygen supply and activates signalling pathways relevant to adaptive responses. For example, HIF inhibits stem cells, promotes tumour cell growth and inflammatory processes. Furthermore, in addition to the vegetative chronic stress reaction in mask wearers, which is channelled via brain centres, there is also likely to be an adverse influence on metabolism at the cellular level. With the prospect of continued mask use in everyday life, this also opens up an interesting field of research for the future.

The fact that prolonged exposure to latently elevated CO_2 levels and toxic air compositions has disease-promoting effects was recognised in 1983, in what the WHO described as "Sick Building Syndrome" (SBS), a condition in which people living indoors experienced relevant effects that increase with the time of their stay, without other specific causes or diseases. The syndrome affects people who spend most of their time indoors, often with subliminally elevated CO_2 levels, and are prone to symptoms such as increased heart rate, rise in blood pressure, headaches, fatigue and difficulty concentrating. Some of the complaints described in the mask studies we found are surprisingly similar to those of Sick Building Syndrome.

Temperature, carbon dioxide content of the air, headaches, dizziness, drowsiness and itching also play a role in Sick Building Syndrome. On the one hand, masks could themselves be responsible for effects such as those described for Sick Building Syndrome when used for a longer period of time. On the other hand, they could additionally intensify these effects when worn in air-conditioned buildings, especially when masks are mandatory indoors.

Many studies show significant clinical relevance and evidence of heart rate increase, headache, fatigue and concentration problems associated with mask wearing.

According to the scientific results and findings, the effects described in healthy people are all more pronounced in sick people, since their compensatory mechanisms, depending on the severity of the illness, are reduced or even non-existing. The relevance of symptoms is also likely to increase with the duration of use.

Further research is needed to shed light on the long-term consequences of widespread mask use in relation to hypoxia and hypercapnia in the general population, also regarding possible exacerbating effects on cardiorespiratory lifestyle diseases such as hypertension, sleep apnoea and metabolic syndrome.

The already often elevated blood carbon dioxide (CO_2) levels in overweight people, sleep apnoea patients and patients with overlap-COPD could possibly increase even further. For such patients, hypercapnia means an increase in the risk of serious diseases with increased morbidity, which could then be further increased by excessive mask use.

Negative physical and psychological changes caused by masks could be objectified even in younger and healthy individuals. The scientifically repeatedly measurable physical and chemical effects were often accompanied by typical subjective complaints and pathophysiological phenomena.

Significant physiological, psychological, somatic and general pathological changes and their frequent occurrence proved a statistically significant correlation with fatigue and oxygen depletion under mask use. In the German study *Is a Mask That Covers the Mouth and Nose Free from Undesirable Side Effects in Everyday Use and Free of Potential Hazards?* there was a combined occurrence of the physical parameter of temperature rise under the mask with the symptom of respiratory impairment in seven of the nine studies concerned (88%). A similar result was shown for the decrease in oxygen saturation under the mask and the symptom of respiratory impairment with detection in six of the eight studies concerned (67%). A combined occurrence of carbon dioxide rise under N95 mask use in nine of the eleven scientific papers (82%). Oxygen drop under N95 mask use with simultaneous co-occurrence in eight of the eleven primary papers (72%). The use of N95 masks was also associated with headache in six of the 10 primary studies concerned (60%). A combined occurrence of the physical parameters of temperature rise and humidity under masks was found in six of the six studies (100%) with significant high results.

Since the symptoms were described in combination in mask wearers and were not observed in isolation in the majority of the cases, the German study refers to them as general Mask-Induced Exhaustion Syndrome (MIES) because of the consistent presentation in numerous papers from different disciplines.

It is also important to notice that in most scientific studies, the exposure time to masks in the context of the measurements and investigations was significantly less than what is expected of workers and the general public under the current regulations and mandates.

The above considerations lead to the conclusion that the negative effects of masks, especially in some individuals and the very elderly, may well be more severe and adverse with prolonged use than presented in some mask studies.

It may also be difficult to assess children and adults who, due to social pressure to wear a mask and the desire to feel they belong, suppress their own needs and concerns until the effects of masks have a noticeable negative impact on their health. The use of masks should be stopped immediately at least when shortness of breath, dizziness or vertigo occur.

Elderly, high-risk patients with lung disease, cardiac patients, pregnant women and stroke patients should be advised to consult a doctor to discuss the safety of masks as their lung volume or cardiopulmonary performance may be reduced and considering that a correlation between age, vulnerable individuals and the occurrence of the aforementioned symptoms while wearing a mask has been statistically proven. Patients with reduced cardiopulmonary function are at increased risk of developing serious respiratory failure with mask use according to the referenced literature. Without the possibility of continuous medical monitoring, it can be concluded that they should not wear masks without close monitoring. The American Asthma and Allergy Society has already advised caution in the use of masks with regard to the COVID-19 pandemic for people with moderate and severe lung disease. Since the severely overweight, sleep apnoea patients and overlap-COPD sufferers are known to be prone to hypercapnia, they also represent a risk group for serious adverse health effects under extensive mask use. This is because the potential of masks to produce additional CO_2 retention may not only have a disruptive effect on the blood gases and respiratory physiology of sufferers, but may also lead to further serious adverse health effects in the long term. Interestingly, in an animal experiment an increase in CO_2 with hypercapnia leads to contraction of smooth airway muscles with constriction of the bronchi. This effect could explain the observed pulmonary decompensation of patients with lung disease under masks.

Patients with renal insufficiency requiring dialysis are, according to the literature available, further candidates for a possible exemption from the mask requirement.

Since it can be assumed that children react even more sensitively to masks, the literature suggests that masks are a contraindication for children with epilepsies (hyperventilation is a trigger for seizures). In the field of paediatrics, special attention should also be paid to the mask symptoms described under psychological, psychiatric and sociological effects with possible triggering of panic attacks by CO_2 rebreathing in the case of predisposition and also reinforcement of claustrophobic fears. The mask-related disturbance of verbal and non-verbal communication and, consequently, of social interaction is particularly serious for children. Masks restrict social interaction and block positive perceptions, smiling, laughing and emotional mimicry.

The proven mask-induced, mild to moderate cognitive impairment with compromised thinking, decreased attention and dizziness, as well as the psychological and neurological effects, should be additionally taken into account when masks are compulsory at school and in both public and non-public transport, also regarding the possibility of an increased risk of incidents.

The long-term sociological, psychological and educational consequences of a comprehensive masking requirement extended to schools are also unpredictable with regard to the psychological and physical development of healthy children. It is worth considering that, according to the Corona Thesis Paper of the University of Bremen, children "are infected less often, they become ill less often, the lethality is close to zero, and they also pass on the infection less often". Other studies show virtually no infections, hardly any mortality and only low contagion in children.

A recent German observational study of 5600 reporting paediatricians also showed a surprisingly low incidence of COVID-19 disease in children. The infection of adults with SARS-CoV-2 by children has been considered in only one suspected case, but could not be proven with certainty, since the parents also had numerous contacts and exposure factors for viral infections due to their occupation.

In this case, the circulating headlines in the public media that children contribute more to the incidence of infection are to be regarded as anecdotal.

In pregnant women, the use of masks during exertion or at rest over long periods of time is to be regarded as critical as little research has been done on this. If there is clear scientific evidence of increased dead space ventilation with possible accumulation of CO_2 in the mother's blood, the use of masks by pregnant women for more than one hour, as well as under physical stress, should be avoided in order to protect the unborn child. The hypercapnia-promoting masks could act as a disruption in the foetal/maternal CO_2 gradient.

According to the literature on psychiatric side effects (personality disorders with anxiety and panic attacks, claustrophobia, dementia and schizophrenia), masking should only be done, if at all, with careful consideration of the advantages and disadvantages. Attention should be paid to possible provocation of the number and severity of panic attacks.

In patients with headaches, a worsening of symptoms can be expected with prolonged mask use. As a result of the increase in blood carbon dioxide (CO_2) when the mask is used, vasodilatation occurs in the central nervous system and the pulsation of the blood vessels decreases. It is also interesting to note radiological experiments that demonstrate an increase in brain volume under sub-threshold, but still within normal limits of CO_2 increase in the blood, observed through structural MRI. The authors interpreted the increase in brain volume as an expression of an increase in blood volume due to a CO_2 increase-induced dilation of the cerebral vessels. The consequences of such sub threshold carbon dioxide (CO_2) increases even under masks are unclear for people with pathological issues inside the skull (aneurysms, tumours, etc.) especially due to longer exposure while wearing a mask, but could be of great relevance due to the blood gas-related volume shifts that take place.

The primary studies often showed weaknesses in the evaluation of cognitive and neuropsychological parameters.

In view of the increased dead space volume, the long-term and increased accumulation and rebreathing of other respiratory air components apart from CO_2 is also relevant, both in children and in old and sick people. Exhaled air contains over 250 substances, including irritant or toxic gases such as nitrogen oxides (NO), hydrogen sulphide (H_2S), isoprene and acetone. Pathological effects and disease have been described in environmental medicine even at a low but chronic exposure to nitrogen oxides and hydrogen sulphide.

Among the volatile organic compounds in exhaled air, acetone and isoprene dominate in terms of quantity, but allyl methyl sulphide, propionic acid and ethanol should also be mentioned. Whether such substances also react chemically with each other underneath masks and in the dead space volume created by masks, and with the mask tissue itself, and in what quantities these and possible reaction products are rebreathed, has not yet been clarified. In addition to the blood gas changes described above (O_2 drop and CO_2 rise), these effects could also play a role with regard to undesirable mask effects. Further research is needed and it is of particular interest in the case of prolonged use of masks.

The WHO promote the production of homemade fabric masks as a potential social and economic benefit. Due to the global shortage of surgical masks and personal protective equipment, it sees this as a source of income and points out that the reuse of fabric masks can reduce costs and waste and contribute to sustainability. In addition to the question of certification procedures for such fabric masks, it should also be mentioned that due to the extensive mask obligation, textile artificial substances in the form of micro- and nanoparticles, some of which cannot be degraded in the body, are chronically absorbed into the body through inhalation to an unusual extent. In the case of medical masks, disposable polymers such as polypropylene, polyurethane, polyacrylonitrile, polystyrene, polycarbonate, polyethylene and polyester should be mentioned.

ENT physicians have already been able to detect such particles in the nasal mucosa of mask wearers causing mucosal reactions and rhinitis. In previous chapters we have also seen that nano plastic has been found in human blood, cells and lungs. In the case of community masks, other substances from the textile industry are likely to be added to those mentioned above. The body will try to absorb these substances through macrophages and scavenger cells in the respiratory tract and alveoli as part of a foreign body reaction.

Toxin release and corresponding local and generalised reactions may occur in case of an unsuccessful attempt to break them down. Extensive use also potentially carries the risk of leading to a mask-related pulmonary or even generalised disorder, as is already known from textile workers chronically exposed to organic dusts in the Third World, likely to contract byssinosis.

For the general public and from a scientific point of view, it is necessary to draw on the long-standing knowledge of respiratory protection in occupational medicine in order to protect children in particular from harm caused by uncertified masks and improper use.

In conclusion, the universal extended mask requirement contradicts the claim of an increased need for individualised medicine with a focus on the unique characteristics of each human being.

Mask research should also set itself the future goal of investigating and defining subgroups for whom respiratory protection use is particularly risky.

Recent studies on SARS-CoV-2 show both a significantly lower infectivity and a significantly lower case mortality than previously assumed. In early October 2020, the WHO also publicly announced that projections show COVID-19 to be fatal for approximately 0.14% of those who become ill compared to 0.10% for endemic influenza, again a figure far lower than expected.

On the other hand, the side effects of masks are clinically relevant.

Both healthy and sick people can experience Mask-Induced Exhaustion Syndrome (MIES), with typical changes and symptoms that are often observed in combination.

A long-term generation of high blood pressure, arteriosclerosis and coronary heart disease and of neurological diseases is scientifically obvious. Extended mask-wearing would have the potential to cause a chronic sympathetic stress response induced by blood gas modifications controlled by brain centres. This in turn induces and triggers immune suppression and metabolic syndrome with cardiovascular and neurological diseases.

There is evidence in the reviewed mask literature of potential long-term effects and also of an increase in direct short-term effects with increased mask-wearing time in terms of cumulative effects for: carbon dioxide retention, drowsiness, headache, feelings of exhaustion, skin irritation (redness, itching) and microbiological contamination (germ colonisation).

Overall, the exact frequency of the described symptom constellation MIES in the mask-using populace remains unclear and cannot be estimated due to insufficient data.

Theoretically, the mask-induced effects also produce increased inflammatory and cancer-promoting effects and can, thus, also have a negative influence on pre-existing clinical pictures.

Further research is particularly desirable in the gynaecological (foetal and embryonic) and paediatric fields, as children are a vulnerable group that would face the longest and most profound consequences of potentially risky mask use. Basic research at the cellular level regarding mask-induced triggering of HIF with potential promotion of immunosuppression and carcinogenicity should also be undertaken.

In any case, the MIES potentially triggered by masks contrasts with the WHO definition of health: "health is a state of complete physical, mental and social well-being and not merely the absence of disease or infirmity."

In addition, to protect the health of their patients, doctors should also base their actions on the guiding principle of the 1948 Geneva Declaration, as revised in 2017. According to this, every doctor vows to put the health and dignity of his patient first and, even under threat, not to use his medical knowledge to violate human rights and civil liberties. This is entirely in accordance with the principles of the Nuremberg Code, evidence-based medicine and the ethical guidelines of clinicians.

In a nutshell, as anticipated in the title of this book, masks are not just useless and detrimental on a 360-degree perspective but with time can also cause severe injuries and death.

APPENDIX

Legislation and your rights in the UK

GDPR & Other Violations: MEDICAL DATA PRIVACY, TRACK & TRACE, MEDICAL TESTING, FACE MASKS, VACCINE PASSPORTS

The Facts:

The General Data Protection Regulation (GDPR - https://gdpr-info.eu/) was first introduced to the UK in May 2018 as EU legislation and on 1st January 2021 became part of UK Law following Brexit.

The Equality Act 2010 (https://www.legislation.gov.uk/ukpga/2010/15/contents) prevents any company introducing policy which could cause discrimination.

The Bribery Act 2010 (https://www.legislation.gov.uk/ukpga/2010/23/section/1) clearly outlines policy including actions demonstrating violation of this law (Blackmail).

High Consequence Infectious Disease (HCID) status in UK - Currently no known HCID's in UK (https://www.gov.uk/guidance/high-consequence-infectious-disease-country-specific-risk#countries-u-to-z)

Health & Safety At Work Act 1974, legal requirement to carry out a Risk

Assessment for a company.

Management of Health & Safety Act 1999, requirements of individual Risk Assessments for all employees and customers (https://www.legislation. gov.uk/uksi/1999/3242/regulation/3/made) Risk Assessment 3, (1) (b) In regards to health reasons this must be carried out by a medical professional at company expense.

As of 19th March 2020, COVID-19 is no longer considered to be a HCID in the UK (https://www.gov.uk/guidance/high-consequence-infectious-diseases-hcid)

A business whether Private or Public must abide by GDPR regulations and the Equality Act 2010 and ignorance of the above laws will not prevent transgressors from being held liable, prosecuted and fined accordingly.

On 13th March 2020, the World Health Organisation (WHO) lowered the risk status of Sars_Cov _2 (Covid-19) to its current status of not being a HCID and the UK also downgraded Covid-19 accordingly on 19th March 2020. To be clear, this means there is no current HCID in the UK.

Unlawful measures and legislation rendering companies liable to prosecution & compensation:

On 24th March 2020, following the advice of SAGE, lockdowns were unlawfully introduced and emergency measures implemented on the basis of a non-existent HCID.

The Coronavirus Act 2020 (https://www.legislation.gov.uk/ukpga/2020/7/ part/1/) was additionally enacted specifically for said HCID and which therefore also has no justification or validity for the aforementioned reasons.

The Health & Safety At Work Act requires a risk assessment before introducing company policy or government guidelines. This will include whether any HCID is in existence in the UK. If not then to select any disease and treatment would be considered an invasion of medical privacy. Thus face masks, Lateral Flow tests (LFT) or PCR tests, Temperature

Checks, Isolation / Quarantine for health reasons attributed to one disease out of many is unlawful, unless decided by a person's GP. There is no substantiated risk to anyone's wellbeing.

GDPR & Other Violations

The Coronavirus Act 2020 required cases of COVID-19 to be reported by a person's GP, but does not allow for random or regular recording of an individual's health records, in part or otherwise, without first establishing the existence of a current HCID. GDPR Article 9 prevents any person or company other than the subjects GP or hospital from processing or storing this data, including any measure supposedly mandated by government.

Under GDPR Article 9, companies are therefore unable to use Article 6, 1(c) & (f) unless they can establish there is a current HCID within the UK.

Recording a name, personal telephone number or any personally identifiable data for health or medical reasons (e.g. the Track & Trace system / Vaccine Passport Verification) is classed as medical data and is thus subject to the restrictions of the use and collection of Special Data as stipulated in Article 9 of the GDPR regulations. In addition to the above any attempt of processing or recording health data would be a violation of the Human Rights legislation Article 8. This also applies to attempting to enforce any restrictions or coerce a person (blackmail) such as wearing face masks, which are harmful due to hypoxia, hypercapnia and other causes.

Finally, people are not obliged to undergo COVID-19 tests in any circumstances or divulge personal medical data based on this, and this is also for a number of reasons.

However, in the first instance, we would like to underline that our right to decline this test is protected under the Nuremberg Code (1947), which clearly stipulates that all medical procedures must have the voluntary informed consent of the human subject.

Nuremberg code Article 6 Section 3, No government can mandate or force medical treatment without individual consent. Therefore, company policy certainly cannot. Including NHS service providers.

This includes any apparatus for health reasons, such as Temperature check, face masks & PCR / lateral flow tests. Additionally forced isolation and quarantine of healthy persons is prohibited.

The intrusive nature of the PCR test is of particular concern and not warranted if the disease can be spread by aerosol. But most importantly and overlooked is the fact the tests are coated in ethylene oxide for sterilising. This is a known cancer causing agent so should not be going anywhere near a person's body.

Conclusion and follow up actions:

Following government guidelines without first establishing a HCID is illegal.

Until such time as the existence of a HCID in the UK can be proven and declared, all companies, organisations and sole traders are therefore prohibited from recording, processing and/or storing Special Data, or attempting to enforce restrictions for unproven health benefit for any reason which is founded upon the alleged existence of a current HCID within the UK.

You are strongly advised to seek legal counsel to verify the above and then make any changes necessary within your business / organisation to ensure that you and/or your company are not held liable for breaches of the aforementioned legislation.

Finally, on 27th May 2022 the government very quietly withdrew all COVID-19 guidelines.
https://www.gov.uk/government/publications/wuhan-novel-coronavirus-infection-prevention-and-   control/new-recommendations-for-primary-and-community-health-care-providers-in-england

REFERENCES

Introduction

En.m.wikipedia.org. (2022). *Wounded healer* - Wikipedia. Available at:

https://en.m.wikipedia.org/wiki/Wounded_healer (Accessed 23/05/2022)

Maineshaman.com. (2022). *What is a wounded healer?* Available at:

https://www.maineshaman.com/blog/category/what-is-a-wounded-healer?format=amp (Accessed 23/05/2022)

Chapter 1

Brief history of breathing

Wildspeak.com (2022). *Introduction to Sacred Breathing*. Available at: http://www.wildspeak.com/other/sacredbreathintro.html (Accessed 28/05/2022)

Williams, E. (2021). *Breathing. An inspired History.* London, United kingdom: Reaktion Books Limited.

eomega.org (2022). *The Healing Power of Breath.* Available at: https://www.eomega.org/article/the-healing-power-of-breath (Accessed 28/05/2022).

Chapter 2

Anatomy and physiology of the respiratory system

Cleveland Clinic (2022). *Respiratory System: Functions, Facts, Organs & Anatomy.* Available at: https://my.clevelandclinic.org/health/articles/21205-respiratory-system (Accessed 07/06/2022).

Lms.rn.com (2022). Available at: https://lms.rn.com/getpdf.php/2048.pdf (Accessed 07/06/2022).

Netafit.org. (2022). Available at: https://www.netafit.org/wp-content/uploads/9232-preview.pdf (Accessed 07/06/2022).

Shier, D., Butler, J. and Lewis, R. (2003). *Hole's essentials of human anatomy and physiology.* Boston: McGraw-Hill.

Graphic design: Pilar Cecilia Montes Bori

Chapter 3

Pranayama, sleeping patterns and other stories

Alzheimer's Society (2022). *Sleep and dementia risk.* Available at: https://www.alzheimers.org.uk/about-dementia/risk-factors-and-prevention/sleep-and-dementia (Accessed 15 June 2022).

Amrit, K., Mahesh, M. (2020). *Effect of oropharyngeal exercise on snoring and quality of sleep among obstructive sleep apnoea patients.* International Journal of Pharmaceutical Research 12(04).

Angermeyer, M., Matschinger, H. (1996). *Public attitude towards psychiatric treatment.* Acta Psychiatrica Scandinavica, 94(5), pp.326-336.

Barth, J., Schumacher, M. and Herrmann-Lingen, C. (2004). *Depression as a Risk Factor for Mortality in Patients With Coronary Heart Disease: A Meta-analysis.* Psychosomatic Medicine. 66(6):802-813.

De Graaf, R., Ten Have, M., Van Gool, C. and Van Dorsselaer, S. (2011).

*Prevalence of mental disorders and trends from 1996 to 2009. Results from the Netherlands Mental Health Survey and Incidence Study-2. Social Psychiatry and Psychiatric Epidemiology.*47(2):203-213.

Carroll, B., Iranmanesh, A., Keenan, D., Cassidy, F., Wilson, W. and Veldhuis, J. (2011). *Pathophysiology of hypercortisolism in depression: pituitary and adrenal responses to low glucocorticoid feedback.* Acta Psychiatrica Scandinavica. 125(6):478-491.

Carson, J., Carson, K., Jones, K., Bennett, R., Wright, C. and Mist, S. (2010). *A pilot randomized controlled trial of the Yoga of Awareness program in the management of fibromyalgia. Pain.* 151(2):530-539.

Cramer, H., Lauche, R., Langhorst, J. and Dobos, G. (2013). *Yoga for depression: A systematic review and meta-analysis. Depression and anxiety.* 30(11):1068-1083.

Hamilton, J. (2020). Available at: https://www.npr.org/sections/health-shots/2020/11/17/935519117/deep-sleep-protects-against-alzheimers-growing-evidence-shows?t=1658405861273 (Accessed 17 June 2022).

Harvard Health (2015). *Too little — or too much — sleep linked to dementia risk - Harvard Health.* Available at: https://www.health.harvard.edu/sleep/too-little-or-too-much-sleep-linked-to-dementia-risk (Accessed 15 June 2022).

Healthline (2022). *How Sleep 'Cleanses' Your Brain and Helps Lower Your Dementia Risk.* Available at: https://www.healthline.com/health-news/how-sleep-cleanses-your-brain-and-helps-lower-your-dementia-risk (Accessed 15 June 2022).

Hoffman, S. and Smits, J. (2008). *Cognitive-Behavioral Therapy for Adult Anxiety Disorders'* The Journal of Clinical Psychiatry. 69(4):621-632.

Hofmann, M., Köhler, B., Leichsenring, F. and Kruse, J. (2013). *Depression as a Risk Factor for Mortality in Individuals with Diabetes: A Meta-Analysis of Prospective Studies.* PLOS ONE. 8(11):p.e79809.

Johnson, N. Hayes, L. Brown, K. Hoo, E. and Ethier, K. (2021). CDC national health report: *Leading causes of morbidity and mortality and associated behavioural risk and protective factors* — United States, 2005–2013.

Lotfalian, S., Spears, C. and Juliano, L. (2020). *The effects of mindfulness-based yogic breathing on craving, affect, and smoking behavior.* Psychology of Addictive Behaviors, 34(2), pp.351-359.

Medeiros, R. Baglietto-Vargas, D. LaFerla, FM. (2010) *The role of tau in Alzheimer's disease and related disorders.* Irvine: Blackwell Publishing Ltd

Nemati, A. (2013). *The effect of pranayama on test anxiety and test performance.* International Journal of Yoga, 6(1), p.55.

NIH (2022). Available at: https://www.nia.nih.gov/health/what-happens-brain-alzheimers-disease (Accessed 17 June 2022).

Pramanik, T., Sharma, H., Mishra, S., Mishra, A., Prajapati, R. and Singh, S. (2009). *Immediate Effect of Slow Pace Bhastrika Pranayama on Blood Pressure and Heart Rate.* The Journal of Alternative and Complementary Medicine, 15(3), pp.293-295.

Pubchem.ncbi.nlm.nih.gov. (2022). Melatonin. Available at:

https://pubchem.ncbi.nlm.nih.gov/compound/Melatonin (Accessed 17 June 2022).

Shahab, L., Sarkar, B. and West, R. (2012). *The acute effects of yogic breathing exercises on craving and withdrawal symptoms in abstaining smokers.* Psychopharmacology, 225(4), pp.875-882.

Shankarappa, V, Prashanti, P., Nachal, A. (2012) Available at: https://www.jcdr.net/articles/PDF/1861/6%20-%203476.(A).pdf (Accessed 21 June 2022).

Sharma, V., Trakroo, M., Subramaniam, V., Sahai, A., Bhavanani, A. and Rajajeyakumar, M. (2013). *Effect of fast and slow pranayama on perceived stress and cardiovascular parameters in young health-care students.* International Journal of Yoga, 6(2), p.104.

Shastri, V., Hankey, A., Sharma, B. and Patra, S. (2017). *Investigation of yoga pranayama and vedic mathematics on mindfulness, aggression and emotion regulation.* International Journal of Yoga, 10(3), p.138.

Shastri, V., Hankey, A., Sharma, B. and Patra, S. (2017). *Investigation of yoga pranayama and Vedic mathematics on mindfulness, aggression and emotion regulation.* International Journal of Yoga, 10(3), p.138.

Stacks.cdc.gov. Available at: https://stacks.cdc.gov/view/cdc/25809 (Accessed 19/11 2021).

Streeter, C., Whitfield, T., Owen, L., Rein, T., Karri, S., Yakhkind, A., Perlmutter, R., Prescot, A., Renshaw, P., Ciraulo, D. and Jensen, J. (2010). *Effects of Yoga Versus Walking on Mood, Anxiety, and Brain GABA Levels: A Randomized Controlled MRS Study.* The Journal of Alternative and Complementary Medicine.16(11):1145-1152.

Subramanian, S. (2014). *Effect of Fast and Slow Pranayama Practice on Cognitive Functions in Healthy Volunteers.* Journal Of Clinical And Diagnostic Research.

Sullivan, C. (2020). *Pranayama Benefits for Physical and Emotional Health.* Available at: https://www.healthline.com/health/pranayama-benefits (Accessed 21 June 2022).

Tiwari, S., Dutt, K., Kumar, R., Dhananjai, S. and Sadashiv, (2013). *Reducing psychological distress and obesity through Yoga practice. International Journal of Yoga.* 6(1):66.

Vedamurthachar, A., Janakiramaiah, N., Hedge, J., Shetty, T., Subbhakrishna, D., Sureshbabu, S. and Gangadhar, B. (2006). *Antidepressant efficacy and hormonal effects of Sudarshana Kriya Yoga (SKY) in alcohol dependent individuals.* Journal of Affective Disorders. 94(1-3):249-253.

Wittchen, H. (2002). *Generalized anxiety disorder: prevalence, burden, and cost to society. Depression and Anxiety.* 16(4):162-171.

Graphic design: Pilar Cecilia Montes Bori

Melatonin image: Pubchem.ncbi.nlm.nih.gov. (2022). Melatonin. Available at:

https://pubchem.ncbi.nlm.nih.gov/compound/Melatonin (Accessed 17 June 2022).

Chapter 4

Masks and peer reviewed articles

Abaluck, J., Kwong, L., Styczynski, A., Haque, A., Kabir, M., Bates-Jefferys, E., Crawford, E., Benjamin-Chung, J., Raihan, S., Rahman, S., Benhachmi, S., Bintee, N., Winch, P., Hossain, M., Reza, H., Jaber, A., Momen, S., Rahman, A., Banti, F., Huq, T., Luby, S. and Mobarak, A. (2022). *Impact of community masking on COVID-19: A cluster-randomized trial in Bangladesh*. Science, 375(6577).

Beder A, Büyükkoçak U, Sabuncuoğlu H, Keskil ZA, Keskil S. (2008) *Preliminary report on surgical mask induced deoxygenation during major surgery*. Neurocirugia (Astur). 19(2):121-6.

Jones, W. (2022). *Face Masks Lead to Breathing Dangerous Levels of Carbon Dioxide Even When Sitting Still, Study Finds*. The Daily Sceptic. Available at: https://dailysceptic.org/2022/05/13/face-masks-lead-to-breathing-dangerous-levels-of-carbon-dioxide-even-when-sitting-still-study-finds/ (Accessed 19 June 2022).

Kisielinski, K., Giboni, P., Prescher, A., Klosterhalfen, B., Graessel, D., Funken, S., Kempski, O. and Hirsch, O. (2021). *Is a Mask That Covers the Mouth and Nose Free from Undesirable Side Effects in Everyday Use and Free of Potential Hazards?*. International Journal of Environmental Research and Public Health, 18(8), p.4344.

LifeSite (2022). *Study supporting alleged mask efficacy excludes key data, risks* - LifeSite. Available at: https://www.lifesitenews.com/opinion/study-supporting-alleged-mask-efficacy-excludes-key-data-risks/ (Accessed 21 June 2022).

Martellucci, C., Flacco, M., Martellucci, M., Violante, F. and Manzoli, L. (2022). *Inhaled CO_2 concentration while wearing face masks: a pilot study using capnography*. Available at: Inhaled CO_2 concentration while wearing face masks: a pilot study using capnography | medRxiv (Accessed 19 June 2022).

End of chapter image adapted from figure 4 in: Kisielinski, K., Giboni, P., Prescher, A., Klosterhalfen, B., Graessel, D., Funken, S., Kempski, O. and Hirsch, O. (2021). *Is a Mask That Covers the Mouth and Nose Free from Undesirable Side Effects in Everyday Use and Free of Potential Hazards?*. International Journal of Environmental Research and Public Health, 18(8), p.4344.

Chapter 5

Masks: physical harm

Agresti, J. D. (2022). *Everything You Always Wanted to Know About Masks, and the Deadly Falsehoods Surrounding Them – Just Facts*. Justfacts. com. Available at: https://www.justfacts.com/news_face_masks_deadly_ falsehoods#harms (Accessed 29 June 2022).

Alexander, P. (2021). *More than 150 Comparative Studies and Articles on Mask Ineffectiveness and Harms* - Brownstone Institute. Brownstone Institute. Available at: https://brownstone.org/articles/more-than-150-comparative-studies-and-articles-on-mask-ineffectiveness-and-harms/ (Accessed 01 July 2022).

Beder, A., Buyukkocak, U., Sabuncuoglu, H., Keskil, Z. and Keskil, S. (2008). *Preliminary report on surgical mask induced deoxygenation during major surgery*. Neurocirugía, 19(2).

Bin-Reza, F., Lopez Chavarrias, V., Nicoll, A. and Chamberland, M. (2011). *The use of masks and respirators to prevent transmission of influenza: a systematic review of the scientific evidence*. Influenza and Other Respiratory Viruses, 6(4), pp.257-267.

Butz, U. Rückatmung von Kohlendioxid bei Verwendung von

Operationsmasken als hygienischer Mundschutz an medizinischem Fachpersonal. Ph.D. Thesis, Fakultät für Medizin der Technischen Universität München, Munich, Germany, 2005.

Clinicaltrials.gov (2005). *The Physiological Impact of N95 Masks on Medical Staff* - Full Text View - ClinicalTrials.gov. Available at:

https://clinicaltrials.gov/ct2/show/NCT00173017 (Accessed 02 July 2022).

Crew, T., Sidley, G. and Lynch, G. (2022). *A chronic case of mask fever* | Gary Sidley The Critic Magazine. The Critic Magazine. Available at: https://thecritic.co.uk/a-chronic-case-of-mask-fever/ (Accessed 29 June 2022).

Da Zhou, C., Sivathondan, P. and Handa, A. (2015). *Unmasking the surgeons: the evidence base behind the use of facemasks in surgery.* Journal of the Royal Society of Medicine, 108(6), pp.223-228.

Delanghe, L., Cauwenberghs, E., Spacova, I., De Boeck, I., Van Beeck, W., Pepermans, K., Claes, I., Vandenheuvel, D., Verhoeven, V. and Lebeer, S. (2021). *Cotton and Surgical Face Masks in Community Settings: Bacterial Contamination and Face Mask Hygiene.* Frontiers in Medicine, 8.

Edmunds, D. (2020). *Could wearing a mask for long periods be detrimental to health?.* Available at: https://www.jpost.com/health-science/could-wearing-a-mask-for-long-periods-be-detrimental-to-health-628400 (Accessed 01 July 2022).

Elisheva, R. (2020). *Adverse Effects of Prolonged Mask Use among Healthcare Professionals during COVID-19.* Journal of Infectious Diseases and Epidemiology, 6(3).

Epstein, D.; Korytny, A.; Isenberg, Y.; Marcusohn, E.; Zukermann, R.; Bishop, B.; Minha, S.; Raz, A.; Miller, *A. Return to Training in the COVID-19 Era: The Physiological Effects of Face Masks during Exercise.* Scand. J. Med. Sci. Sports 2020.

Fikenzer, S.; Uhe, T.; Lavall, D.; Rudolph, U.; Falz, R.; Busse, M.; Hepp, P.;

Laufs, U. *Effects of Surgical and FFP2/N95 Face Masks on Cardiopulmonary Exercise Capacity.* Clin. Res. Cardiol. 2020, 109, 1522–1530.

Foo, C.C.I.; Goon, A.T.J.; Leow, Y.; Goh, C. *Adverse Skin Reactions to Personal Protective Equipment against Severe Acute Respiratory Syndrome*–a Descriptive Study in Singapore. Contact Dermat. 2006, 55, 291–294.

Gaeta, M. (2020). *Why Masks Do More Harm Than Good* - video. [online] Vimeo. Available at: https://vimeo.com/424254660 (Accessed 03 July 2022).

Haase-Fielitz, A.; Meretz, D.; Gäsert, L.; Butter, C. *Einfluss gängiger Gesichtsmasken auf physiologische Parameter und Belastungsempfinden unter arbeitstypischer körperlicher Anstrengung.* Deutsches Ärzteblatt 2020, 674–675.

Hammond, G., Raddatz, R., Gelskey, D. (1989). *Impact of Atmospheric Dispersion and Transport of Viral Aerosols on the Epidemiology of Influenza.* Clinical Infectious Diseases, 11(3), pp.494-497.

Heow, P. L., De Yun W. (2011). *Objective Assessment of Increase in Breathing Resistance of N95 Respirators on Human Subjects.* The Annals of Occupational Hygiene.

Hua, W.; Zuo, Y.; Wan, R.; Xiong, L.; Tang, J.; Zou, L.; Shu, X.; Li, L. *Short-Term Skin Reactions Following Use of N95 Respirators and Medical Masks.* Contact Dermat. 2020, 83, 115–121.

ImunoMedica Clinic (2021). T*he Mask-Induced Exhaustion Syndrome.* Available at: https://www.imuno-medica.ro/news/The-Mask-Induced-Exhaustion-Syndrome-45

(Accessed 01 July 2022).

Jacobs, J., Ohde, S., Takahashi, O., Tokuda, Y., Omata, F., Fukui, T. (2009). *Use of surgical face masks to reduce the incidence of the common cold among health care workers in Japan: A randomized controlled trial.* American Journal of Infection Control, 37(5), pp.417-419.

Kal, E., Young, W., Ellmers, T. (2020). *Face masks, vision, and risk of falls.* BMJ, p.m4133.

Kao, T.W., Huang, K.C., Huang, Y.L., Tsai, T.J., Hsieh, B.S., Wu, M.S. (2004) *The physiological impact of wearing an N95 mask during hemodialysis as a precaution against SARS in patients with end-stage renal disease.* J Formos Med Assoc.;103(8):624-8.

Kisielinski, K., Giboni, P., Prescher, A., Klosterhalfen, B., Graessel, D., Funken, S., Kempski, O. and Hirsch, O. (2021). *Is a Mask That Covers the Mouth and Nose Free from Undesirable Side Effects in Everyday Use and Free of Potential Hazards?.* International Journal of Environmental Research and Public Health, 18(8), p.4344.

Kyung, S.Y.; Kim, Y.; Hwang, H.; Park, J.-W.; Jeong, S.H. *Risks of N95 Face Mask Use in Subjects with COPD.* Respir. Care 2020, 65, 658–664.

Leung, N., Chu, D., Shiu, E., Chan, K., McDevitt, J., Hau, B., Yen, H., Li, Y., Ip, D., Peiris, J., Seto, W., Leung, G., Milton, D., Cowling, B. (2020). *Respiratory virus shedding in exhaled breath and efficacy of face masks.* Nature Medicine, 26(5), pp.676-680.

Li, Y.; Tokura, H.; Guo, Y.P.; Wong, A.S.W.; Wong, T.; Chung, J.; Newton, E. *Effects of Wearing N95 and Surgical Facemasks on Heart Rate, Thermal Stress and Subjective Sensations.* Int. Arch. Occup. Environ. Health 2005, 78, 501–509.

LifeSite (2021). *47 studies confirm ineffectiveness of masks for COVID and 32 more confirm their negative health effects - LifeSite.* Available at: https://www.lifesitenews.com/news/47-studies-confirm-inefectiveness-of-masks-for-covid-and-32-more-confirm-their-negative-health-effects/ (Accessed 02 July 2022).

Lin, T., Tang, F., Hung, P., Hua, Z. and Lai, C. (2018). *Relative survival of Bacillus subtilis spores loaded on filtering facepiece respirators after five decontamination methods.* Indoor Air, 28(5), pp.754-762.

Liu, C.; Li, G.; He, Y.; Zhang, Z.; Ding, Y. *Effects of Wearing Masks on*

Human Health and Comfort during the COVID-19 Pandemic. IOP Conf. Ser. Earth Environ. Sci. 2020, 531, 012034.

MacIntyre, C., Seale, H., Dung, T., Hien, N., Nga, P., Chughtai, A., Rahman, B., Dwyer, D. and Wang, Q. (2015). *A cluster randomised trial of cloth masks compared with medical masks in healthcare workers.* BMJ Open, 5(4), pp.e006577-e006577.

Offeddu, V., Yung, C., Low, M., Tam, C. (2017). *Effectiveness of Masks and Respirators Against Respiratory Infections in Healthcare Workers:* A Systematic Review and Meta-Analysis. Clinical Infectious Diseases, 65(11), pp.1934-1942.

Ong, J.J.Y.; Bharatendu, C.; Goh, Y.; Tang, J.Z.Y.; Sooi, K.W.X.; Tan, Y.L.; Tan, B.Y.Q.; Teoh, H.-L.; Ong, S.T.; Allen, D.M.; et al. *Headaches AssociatedWith Personal Protective Equipment-A Cross-Sectional Study among Frontline Healthcare Workers During COVID-19.* Headache 2020, 60, 864–877

PANDA (2022). *PANDA InfoBank: Masks.* Available at: https://www.pandata.org/infobank-masks/ (Accessed 01 July 2022).

Pifarré, F.; Zabala, D.D.; Grazioli, G.; de Yzaguirre i Maura, I. *COVID 19 and Mask in Sports.* Apunt. Sports Med. 2020.

Principia Scientific Intl. A science-based community. (2021). *65 Studies Reveals Face Masks DO Cause Physical Harm* | Principia Scientific Intl. Available at: https://principia-scientific.com/65-studies-reveals-face-masks-do-cause-physical-harm/ (Accessed 01 July 2022).

Radonovich, L., Simberkoff, M., Bessesen, M., Brown, A., Cummings, D., Gaydos, C., Los, J., Krosche, A., Gibert, C., Gorse, G., Nyquist, A., Reich, N., Rodriguez-Barradas, M., Price, C. and Perl, T. (2019). *N95 Respirators vs Medical Masks for Preventing Influenza Among Health Care Personnel.* JAMA, 322(9), p.824.

Rebmann, T.; Carrico, R.; Wang, J. *Physiologic and Other Effects and Compliance with Long-Term Respirator Use among Medical Intensive Care*

Unit Nurses. Am. J. Infect. Control 2013, 41, 1218–1223.

Rengasamy, S., Eimer, B., Shaffer, R. (2010). *Simple Respiratory Protection—Evaluation of the Filtration Performance of Cloth Masks and Common Fabric Materials Against 20–1000 nm Size Particles.* The Annals of Occupational Hygiene.

Roberge, R.J.; Kim, J.-H.; Powell, J.B. *N95 Respirator Use during Advanced Pregnancy.* Am. J. Infect. Control 2014, 42, 1097–1100.

Roberge, R.; Bayer, E.; Powell, J.; Coca, A.; Roberge, M.; Benson, S. *Effect of Exhaled Moisture on Breathing Resistance of N95 Filtering Facepiece Respirators.* Ann. Occup. Hyg. 2010, 54, 671–677.

Roberge, R.J.; Kim, J.-H.; Benson, S.M. *Absence of Consequential Changes in Physiological, Thermal and Subjective Responses from Wearing a Surgical Mask.* Respir. Physiol. Neurobiol. 2012, 181, 29–35.

Rosner, E. *Adverse Effects of Prolonged Mask Use among Healthcare Professionals during COVID-19.* J. Infect. Dis. Epidemiol. 2020.

Shakya, K., Noyes, A., Kallin, R. and Peltier, R. (2016. *Evaluating the efficacy of cloth facemasks in reducing particulate matter exposure.* Journal of Exposure Science & Environmental Epidemiology, 27(3), pp.352-357.

Sinkule, E., Powell, J., Goss, F. (2012). *Evaluation of N95 Respirator Use with a Surgical Mask Cover: Effects on Breathing Resistance and Inhaled Carbon Dioxide.* The Annals of Occupational Hygiene.

Smith, J., MacDougall, C., Johnstone, J., Copes, R., Schwartz, B., Garber, G. (2016). *Effectiveness of N95 respirators versus surgical masks in protecting health care workers from acute respiratory infection: a systematic review and meta-analysis.* Canadian Medical Association Journal, 188(8), pp.567-574.

Spooner, J. (1967). *History of Surgical Face Masks.* AORN Journal, 5(1), pp.76-80.

Swiss Policy Research (2021). *The Face Mask Folly in Retrospect.* Available at: https://swprs.org/the-face-mask-folly-in-retrospect/ (Accessed 01 July 2022).

Swiss Policy Research (2022). *Are Face Masks Effective? The Evidence.* Available at: https://swprs.org/face-masks-and-covid-the-evidence/ (Accessed 01 July 2022).

TheBlaze (2022). *Horowitz: The danger of the momentum behind N95 respirators.* Available at: https://www.theblaze.com/op-ed/horowitz-the-danger-of-the-momentum-behind-n95-respirators (Accessed 02 July 2022).

Van Vuuren, F.,(2021). *Coronavirus masks are killing people, dentists warn.* Linkedin.com. Available at: https://www.linkedin.com/pulse/coronavirus-masks-killing-people-dentists-warn-fanie-van-vuuren (Accessed 29 June 2022).

WHO (2020) *Advice on the use of masks in the context of COVID-19 - Interim guidance.* Available at: WHO-2019-nCov-IPC_Masks-2020.4-eng.pdf (Accessed 21 June 2022).

Wong, C.K.M.; Yip, B.H.K.; Mercer, S.; Griffiths, S.; Kung, K.;Wong, M.C.; Chor, J.;Wong, S.Y. *Effect of Facemasks on Empathy and Relational Continuity: A Randomised Controlled Trial in Primary Care.* BMC Fam. Pract. 2013, 14, 200.

Yezli, S., Otter, J. (2011). *Minimum Infective Dose of the Major Human Respiratory and Enteric Viruses Transmitted Through Food and the Environment.* Food and Environmental Virology, 3(1), pp.1-30.

Picture: Alice Motola

Chapter 6

The expert's view

Horowitz, D. (2022). Conservative Review with Daniel Horowitz: Ep

826 | *Only a Neanderthal Can Believe a Mask Stops a Virus* | Guest: Stephen Petty on Apple Podcasts. Apple Podcasts. Available at: https://podcasts. apple.com/us/podcast/ep-826-only-a-neanderthal-can-believe-a-mask/ id1065050908?i=1000511752553 (Accessed 05 July 2022).

Showmeyoursmile.org (2021). *Interview with Industrial Hygienist Stephen Petty on Masks as an exposure control* - Showmeyoursmile.org. Available at: https://showmeyoursmile.org/interviews/mitigation-and-masks/ (Accessed 05 July 2022).

Youtube.com (2021). Available at: https://www.youtube.com/ watch?v=oYEo4T6V25w (Accessed 05 July 2022).

Youtube.com (2022). Available at: https://www.youtube.com/ watch?v=J3dnkbKoj4A (Accessed 5 July 2022).

Graphics and diagrams kindly provided by Stephen Petty at EES Group, Inc.

Chapter 7

Masks: emotional and psychological harm

Agresti, D. (2021). *Everything You Always Wanted to Know About Masks, and the Deadly Falsehoods Surrounding Them* – Just Facts. Justfacts.com. Available at: https://www.justfacts.com/news_face_masks_deadly_ falsehoods#harms (Accessed 05 July 2022).

Breton-Provencher, V., Drummond, G., Sur, M. (2021). Locus Coeruleus *Norepinephrine in Learned Behavior: Anatomical Modularity and Spatiotemporal Integration in Targets.* Frontiers in Neural Circuits, 15.

Clinicaltrials.gov (2005). *The Physiological Impact of N95 Masks on Medical Staff* - Full Text View - ClinicalTrials.gov. Available at:

https://clinicaltrials.gov/ct2/show/NCT00173017 (Accessed 07 July 2022).

Crew, T., Sidley, G., Lynch, G. (2022). *A chronic case of mask fever.* The Critic Magazine. The Critic Magazine. Available at: https://thecritic. co.uk/a-chronic-case-of-mask-fever/ (Accessed 07 July 2022).

Hart group (2022). Available at: https://www.hartgroup.org/healthcare-venues-persisting-masks/ (Accessed 07 July 2022).

Hearing Link Services (2022). *Deafness & hearing loss facts* - Hearing Link Services. Available at: https://www.hearinglink.org/your-hearing/about-hearing/facts-about-deafness-hearing-loss/ (Accessed 07 July 2022).

Kung, S., Shen, Y., Chang, E., Hong, Y., Wang, L. (2018). *Hypercapnia impaired cognitive and memory functions in obese patients with obstructive sleep apnoea.* Scientific Reports, 8(1).

Norcross, J.C. [Ed] (2011). *Psychotherapy relationships that work.* 2nd edition. New York. Oxford University Press

Smile Free (2022). Harms - Smile Free. Available at: https://smilefree.org/harms/ (Accessed 07 July 2022).

Zheng, G., Wang, Y., Wang, X. (2008). *Chronic hypoxia-hypercapnia influences cognitive function: A possible new model of cognitive dysfunction in chronic obstructive pulmonary disease.* Medical Hypotheses, 71(1), pp.111-113.

Chapter 8

Masks: environmental harm

Brown, A. (2022). *Study finds plastics found in masks present in patients' lungs.* Western Standard. Available at: https://www.westernstandard.news/features/study-finds-plastics-found-in-masks-present-in-patients-lungs/article_056590f2-0615-5bc9-aab0-730e7704634e.html (Accessed 11 July 2022).

Carrington, D. (2022). *Microplastics found in human blood for first time.* The Guardian. Available at: https://www.theguardian.com/

environment/2022/mar/24/microplastics-found-in-human-blood-for-first-time (Accessed 17 July 2022).

Carrington, D. (2022). *Microplastics cause damage to human cells, study shows.* The Guardian. Available at:

https://www.theguardian.com/environment/2021/dec/08/microplastics-damage-human-cells-study-plastic (Accessed 17 July 2022).

Corbyn, P. (2022). *Man-Made Climate Change Does not Exist!* Reading University Debating Journal. Available at:

https://readingunidebating.wordpress.com/2019/09/19/piers-corbyn-man-made-climate-change-does-not-exist/ (Accessed 17 July 2022).

Danopoulos, E., Twiddy, M., West, R., Rotchell, J. (2022). *A rapid review and meta-regression analyses of the toxicological impacts of microplastic exposure in human cells.* Journal of Hazardous Materials, 427, p.127861.

Fleury, J., Baulin, V. (2021). *Microplastics destabilize lipid membranes by mechanical stretching.* Proceedings of the National Academy of Sciences, 118(31).

Gruber, E., Stadlbauer, V., Pichler, V., Resch-Fauster, K., Todorovic, A., Meisel, T., Trawoeger, S., Hollóczki, O., Turner, S., Wadsak, W., Vethaak, A., Kenner, L. (2022). *To Waste or Not to Waste: Questioning Potential Health Risks of Micro- and Nanoplastics with a Focus on Their Ingestion and Potential arcinogenicity.* Exposure and Health.

Jenner, L., Rotchell, J., Bennett, R., Cowen, M., Tentzeris, V., Sadofsky, L. (2022). *Detection of microplastics in human lung tissue using μFTIR spectroscopy.* Science of The Total Environment, 831, p.154907.

Leslie, H., van Velzen, M., Brandsma, S., Vethaak, A., Garcia-Vallejo, J., Lamoree, M. (2022). *Discovery and quantification of plastic particle pollution in human blood.* Environment International, 163, p.107199.

Li, L., Zhao, X., Li, Z.,Song, K. (2021). *COVID-19: Performance study of microplastic inhalation risk posed by wearing masks.* Journal of Hazardous

Materials, 411, p.124955.

Poudel, S. (2021). *Disposing of face masks: The next environmental problem?*. Unicef.org. Available at: https://www.unicef.org/nepal/stories/disposing-face-masks-next-environmental-problem (Accessed 09 July 2022).

Ragusa, A., Svelato, A., Santacroce, C., Catalano, P., Notarstefano, V., Carnevali, O., Papa, F., Rongioletti, M., Baiocco, F., Draghi, S., D'Amore, E., Rinaldo, D., Matta, M., Giorgini, E. (2021). *Plasticenta: First evidence of microplastics in human placenta.* Environment International, 146, p.106274.

Roberts, K., Bowyer, C., Kolstoe, S., Fletcher, S. (2022). *Coronavirus face masks: an environmental disaster that might last generations.* The Conversation. Available at: https://theconversation.com/coronavirus-face-masks-an-environmental-disaster-that-might-last-generations-144328 (Accessed 09 July 2022).

Robinson, A.B., Robinson, N.E., Soon, W. (2022). Global Warming Petition Project. Petitionproject.org. Available at:

http://www.petitionproject.org/gw_article/Review_Article_HTML.php (Accessed 17 July 2022).

Shiferie, F. (2021). *Improper disposal of face masks during COVID-19: unheeded public health threat.* Pan African Medical Journal, 38.

UN News (2022). *Five things you should know about disposable masks and plastic pollution.* Available at: https://news.un.org/en/story/2020/07/1069151 (Accessed 09 July 2022).

World Economic Forum (2020). *How face masks, gloves and other coronavirus waste is polluting our ocean.* Available at: https://www.weforum.org/agenda/2020/06/ppe-masks-gloves-coronavirus-ocean-pollution/ (Accessed 11 July 2022).

Drawing: Lucia Isabella Carla Bruno

Diagrams and graphics:

Corbyn, P. (2022). *Man-Made Climate Change Does not Exist!* Reading University Debating Journal. Available at:

https://readingunidebating.wordpress.com/2019/09/19/piers-corbyn-man-made-climate-change-does-not-exist/ (Accessed 17 July 2022).

Robinson, A.B., Robinson, N.E., Soon, W. (2022). *Global Warming Petition Project.* Petitionproject.org. Available at:

http://www.petitionproject.org/gw_article/Review_Article_HTML.php (Accessed 17 July 2022).

Chapter 9

Masks: harm to Children

Breitbart (2022). *Die COVID-19 Pandemie und Lesekompetenz von Viertklässler*innen:* Ergebnisse der IFS-Schulpanelstudie 2016-2021. TU Dortmund. Available at: https://ifs.ep.tu-dortmund.de/details/die-covid-19-pandemie-und-lesekompetenz-von-viertklaesslerinnen-ergebnisse-der-ifs-schulpanelstudie-2016-2021-18640/ (Accessed 27 August 2022).

Bridle, B., 2021. *Un an de restrictions sanitaires augmente les risques d'allergies, d'asthme et de maladies auto-immunes chez les enfants.* The Conversation. Available at: https://theconversation.com/un-an-de-restrictions-sanitaires-augmente-les-risques-dallergies-dasthme-et-de-maladies-auto-immunes-chez-les-enfants-156898

(Accessed 19 July 2022).

Bridle, D. (2022). *Stop Masking Children.* Viralimmunologist.substack.com. Available at: https://viralimmunologist.substack.com/p/stop-masking-children?s=r (Accessed 19 July 2022).

Dyer, O. (2022). *Covid-19: Children born during the pandemic score lower on cognitive tests, study finds.* BMJ, p.n2031.

Hill, M. (2022). *School Mask Mandates Mean Trauma For Millions*

Of Children, Especially Those From Low-Income Families | From the Trenches World Report. From the Trenches World Report. Available at: https://fromthetrenchesworldreport.com/school-mask-mandates-mean-trauma-for-millions-of-children-especially-those-from-low-income-families/290974 (Accessed 27 August 2022).

Ludvigsson, J., Engerström, L., Nordenhäll, C., Larsson, E. (2021). *Open Schools, Covid-19, and Child and Teacher Morbidity in Sweden.* New England Journal of Medicine, 384(7), pp.669-671.

Ofstead (2022). *Education recovery in early years providers: summer 2022.* GOV.UK. Available at: https://www.gov.uk/government/publications/education-recovery-in-early-years-providers-summer-2022 (Accessed 27 August 2022)

Powe, A. (2022). *CNN Medical Analyst Who Wanted To Ban The Unvaccinated From Society And Force Children To Mask Now Reveals How Masking Has Severely Harmed Her Son.* The Gateway Pundit. Available at: https://www.thegatewaypundit.com/2022/08/cnn-medical-analyst-wanted-ban-unvaccinated-society-force-children-mask-take-pcr-tests-weekly-attend-school-reveals-masks-wearing-harmed-son/ (Accessed 27 August 2022)

Schwarz, S., Jenetzky, E., Krafft, H., Maurer, T., Martin, D. (2022). *Corona children studies "Co-Ki": First results of a Germany-wide registry on mouth and nose covering (mask) in children.* Available at: https://www.researchsquare.com/article/rs-124394/v3 (Accessed 19 July 2022).

Graphic design: Pilar Cecilia Montes Bori

Chapter 10

Masks and dementia care

American Psychiatric Association (2013). *Diagnostic and Statistical Manual of Mental Disorders,* 5th Edn. Arlington, VA: American Psychiatric Publishing.

Baron-Cohen, S., Wheelwright, S., Hill, J., Raste, Y., and Plumb, I. (2001). *The "Reading the Mind in the Eyes" test revised version: a study with normal adults, and adults with Asperger syndrome or high-functioning autism.* J. Child. Psychol. Psych. Allied Discip. 42, 241–251. doi: 10.1111/1469-7610.00715

Benussi, A., Premi, E., Gazzina, S., Brattini, C., Bonomi, E., Alberici, A., et al. (2021). *Progression of behavioral disturbances and neuropsychiatric symptoms in patients with genetic frontotemporal dementia.* JAMA Netw. Open 4:e2030194.

Bisenius, S., Neumann, J., and Schroeter, M. L. (2016). *Validating new diagnostic imaging criteria for primary progressive aphasia via anatomical likelihood estimation meta-analyses.* Eur. J. Neurol. 23, 704–712. doi: 10.1111/ene.12902

Bora, E., Walterfang, M., and Velakoulis, D. (2015). *Theory of mind in behavioural-variant frontotemporal dementia and Alzheimer's disease: a meta-analysis.* J. Neurol. Neurosurg. Psychiatry 86, 714–719. doi: 10.1136/jnnp-2014-309445

Bora, E., and Yener, G. G. (2017). *Meta-analysis of social cognition in mild cognitive impairment.* J. Geriatr. Psychiatry Neurol. 30, 206–213. doi: 10.1177/0891988717710337

Carbon, C. C. (2020). *Wearing face masks strongly confuses counterparts in reading emotions.* Front. Psychol. 11:566886. doi: 10.3389/fpsyg.2020.566886

Cartaud, A., Quesque, F., and Coello, Y. (2020). *Wearing a face mask against Covid-19 results in a reduction of social distancing.* PLoS ONE 15:e0243023. doi: 10.1371/journal.pone.0243023

Cerami, C., Santi, G. C., Galandra, C., Dodich, A., Cappa, S. F., Vecchi, T., et al. (2020). *Covid-19 outbreak in Italy: are we ready for the psychosocial and the economic crisis?* Baseline findings from the PsyCovid study. Front. Psychiatry 11:556. doi: 10.3389/fpsyt.2020.00556

Chaby, L., Hupont, I., Avril, M., Luherne-du Boullay, V., and Chetouani, M. (2017). *Gaze behavior consistency among older and younger adults when looking at emotional faces.* Front. Psychol. 8:548. doi: 10.3389/fpsyg.2017.00548

Chen, N., Zhou, M., Dong, X., Qu, J., Gong, F., Han, Y., et al. (2020). *Epidemiological and clinical characteristics of 99 cases of 2019 novel coronavirus pneumonia in Wuhan, China: a descriptive study.* Lancet 395, 507–513. doi: 10.1016/S0140-6736(20)30211-7

Chern, A., and Golub, J. S. (2019). *Age-related hearing loss and dementia.* Alzheimer Dis. Assoc. Disord. 33, 285–290. doi: 10.1097/WAD.0000000000000325

Dodich, A., Crespi, C., Santi, G. C., Cappa, S. F., and Cerami, C. (2021). *Evaluation of discriminative detection abilities of social cognition measures for the diagnosis of the behavioral variant of frontotemporal dementia: a systematic review.* Neuropsychol. Rev. 31, 251–266. doi: 10.1007/s11065-020-09457-1

Ebner, N. C., Riediger, M., and Lindenberger, U. (2010). *FACES - A database of facial expressions in young, middle-aged, and older women and men: Development and validation.* Behav. Res. Methods 42, 351–362. doi: 10.3758/BRM.42.1.351

Gorno-Tempini, M. L., Hillis, A. E., Weintraub, S., Kertesz, A., Mendez, M., Cappa, S. F., et al. (2011). *Classification of primary progressive aphasia and its variants.* Neurology 76, 1006–1014. doi: 10.1212/WNL.0b013e31821103e6

Grainger, S. A., and Henry, J. D. (2020). *Gaze patterns to emotional faces throughout the adult lifespan.* Psychol. Aging 35, 981–992. doi: 10.1037/pag0000571

Greenhalgh, T., Schmid, M. B., Czypionka, T., Bassler, D., and Gruer, L. (2020). *Face masks for the public during the covid-19 crisis.* BMJ 369:m1435. doi: 10.1136/bmj.m1435

Hayes, G. S., McLennan, S. N., Henry, J. D., Phillips, L. H., Terrett, G., Rendell, P. G., et al. (2020). *Task characteristics influence facial emotion recognition age-effects: a meta-analytic review.* Psychol. Aging 35, 295–315. doi: 10.1037/pag0000441

Henry, J. D., Phillips, L. H., Ruffman, T., and Bailey, P. E. (2013). *A meta-analytic review of age differences in theory of mind.* Psychol. Aging 28, 826–839. doi: 10.1037/a0030677

Holmes, E. A., O'Connor, R. C., Perry, V. H., Tracey, I., Wessely, S., Arseneault, L., et al. (2020). *Multidisciplinary research priorities for the COVID-19 pandemic: a call for action for mental health science.* Lancet Psychiat. 7, 547–560. doi: 10.1016/S2215-0366(20)30168-1

Jessen, F., Amariglio, R. E., van Boxtel, M., Breteler, M., Ceccaldi, M., Chételat, G., et al. (2014). *A conceptual framework for research on subjective cognitive decline in preclinical Alzheimer's disease.* Alzheimers Dement. 10, 844–852. doi: 10.1016/j.jalz.2014.01.001

Kirkland, R. A., Peterson, E., Baker, C. A., Miller, S., and Pulos, S. (2013). *Meta-analysis reveals adult female superiority in "Reading the Mind in the Eyes" test.* North Am. J. Psychol. 15, 121–146.

Kisielinski, K., Giboni, P., Prescher, A., Klosterhalfen, B., Graessel, D., Funken, S., Kempski, O. and Hirsch, O. (2021). *Is a Mask That Covers the Mouth and Nose Free from Undesirable Side Effects in Everyday Use and Free of Potential Hazards?.* International Journal of Environmental Research and Public Health, 18(8), p.4344.

Kynast, J., Lampe, L., Luck, T., Frisch, S., Arelin, K., Hoffmann, K. T., et al. (2018). *White matter hyperintensities associated with small vessel disease impair social cognition beside attention and memory.* J. Cereb. Blood Flow Metab. 38, 996–1009. doi: 10.1177/0271678X17719380

Kynast, J., Polyakova, M., Quinque, E. M., Hinz, A., Villringer, A., and Schroeter, M. L. (2021). *Age- and sex-specific standard scores for the Reading the Mind in the Eyes test. Front.* Aging Neurosci. 12:607107. doi: 10.3389/fnagi.2020.607107

Kynast, J., Quinque, E. M., Polyakova, M., Luck, T., Riedel-Heller, S. G., Baron-Cohen, S., et al. (2020). *Mindreading from the eyes declines with aging - evidence from 1,603 subjects.* Front. Aging Neurosci. 12:550416. doi: 10.3389/fnagi.2020.550416

Kynast, J., and Schroeter, M. L. (2018). *Sex, age, and emotional valence: revealing possible biases in the 'Reading the Mind in the Eyes' task.* Front. Psychol. 9:570. doi: 10.3389/fpsyg.2018.00570

Lara, E., Martín-María, N., De la Torre-Luque, A., Koyanagi, A., Vancampfort, D., Izquierdo, A., et al. (2019). *Does loneliness contribute to mild cognitive impairment and dementia? A systematic review and meta-analysis of longitudinal studies.* Ageing Res. Rev. 52, 7–16. doi: 10.1016/j.arr.2019.03.002

Maldonado, T., Orr, J. M., Goen, J. R. M., and Bernard, J. A. (2020). *Age differences in the subcomponents of executive functioning.* J. Gerontol. B Psychol. Sci. Soc. Sci. 75, e31–e55. doi: 10.1093/geronb/gbaa005

McKeith, I. G., Boeve, B. F., Dickson, D. W., Halliday, G., Taylor, J. P., Weintraub, D., et al. (2017). *Diagnosis and management of dementia with Lewy bodies: fourth consensus report of the DLB consortium.* Neurology 89, 88–100. doi: 10.1212/WNL.0000000000004058

Mheidly, N., Fares, M. Y., Zalzale, H., and Fares, J. (2020). *Effect of face masks on interpersonal communication during the COVID-19 pandemic.* Front. Public Health 8:582191. doi: 10.3389/fpubh.2020.582191

Mok, V. C. T., Pendlebury, S., Wong, A., Alladi, S., Au, L., Bath, P. M., et al. (2020). *Tackling challenges in care of Alzheimer's disease and other dementias amid the COVID-19 pandemic, now and in the future.* Alzheimers Dement. 16, 1571–1581. doi: 10.1002/alz.12143

Neary, D., Snowden, J. S., Gustafson, L., Passant, U., Stuss, D., Black, S., et al. (1998). *Frontotemporal lobar degeneration: a consensus on clinical diagnostic criteria.* Neurology 51, 1546–1554. doi: 10.1212/WNL.51.6.1546

Pardini, M., Gialloreti, L. E., Mascolo, M., Benassi, F., Abate, L., Guida, S., et al. (2013). *Isolated theory of mind deficits and risk for frontotemporal dementia: a longitudinal pilot study.* J. Neurol. Neurosurg. Psychiatry 84, 818–821. doi: 10.1136/jnnp-2012-303684

Peeples, L. (2020). *What the data say about wearing face masks.* Nature 586, 186–189. doi: 10.1038/d41586-020-02801-8

Pfefferbaum, B., and North, C. S. (2020). *Mental health and the Covid-19 pandemic.* New Engl. J. Med. 383:510–512. doi: 10.1056/NEJMp2008017

Quesque, F., and Rossetti, Y. (2020). *What do theory-of-mind tasks actually measure? Theory and practice.* Perspect. Psychol. Sci. 15, 384–396. doi: 10.1177/1745691619896607

Ruffman, T., Henry, J. D., Livingstone, V., and Phillips, L. H. (2008). *A meta-analytic review of emotion recognition and aging: implications for neuropsychological models of aging.* Neurosci. Biobehav. Rev. 32, 863–881. doi: 10.1016/j.neubiorev.2008.01.001

Santabárbara, J., Villagrasa, B., and Gracia-García, P. (2020). *Does depression increase the risk of dementia?* Updated meta-analysis of prospective studies. Actas Esp. Psiquiatr. 48:169–180.

Schroeter, M. L., Zysset, S., Kruggel, F., and von Cramon, D. Y. (2003). *Age dependency of the hemodynamic response as measured by functional near-infrared spectroscopy.* Neuroimage 19, 555–564. doi: 10.1016/S1053-8119(03)00155-1

Schroeter, M. L., Stein, T., Maslowski, N., and Neumann, J. (2009). *Neural correlates of Alzheimer's disease and mild cognitive impairment: a systematic and quantitative meta-analysis involving 1351 patients.* Neuroimage 47, 1196–1206. doi: 10.1016/j.neuroimage.2009.05.037

Schroeter, M. L., Vogt, B., Frisch, S., Becker, G., Seese, A., Barthel, H., et al. (2011). *Dissociating behavioral disorders in early dementia-an FDG-PET study.* Psychiatry Res. 194, 235–244. doi: 10.1016/j.

pscychresns.2011.06.009

Schroeter, M. L., Vogt, B., Frisch, S., Becker, G., Barthel, H., Mueller, K., et al. (2012). *Executive deficits are related to the inferior frontal junction in early dementia.* Brain 135(Pt 1), 201–215. doi: 10.1093/brain/awr311

Schroeter, M. L., Laird, A. R., Chwiesko, C., Deuschl, C., Schneider, E., Bzdok, D., et al. (2014). *Conceptualizing neuropsychiatric diseases with multimodal data-driven meta-analyses - the case of behavioral variant frontotemporal dementia.* Cortex 57, 22–37. doi: 10.1016/j. cortex.2014.02.022

Schroeter, M. L., Pawelke, S., Bisenius, S., Kynast, J., Schuemberg, K., Polyakova, M., et al. (2018). *A modified reading the mind in the eyes test predicts behavioral variant frontotemporal dementia better than executive function tests.* Front. Aging Neurosci. 10:11. doi: 10.3389/ fnagi.2018.00011

Schroeter, M. L., Albrecht, F., Ballarini, T., Leuthold, D., Legler, A., Hartwig, S., et al. (2020). *Capgras delusion in posterior cortical atrophy - a quantitative multimodal imaging single case study.* Front. Aging Neurosci. 12:133. doi: 10.3389/fnagi.2020.00133

Schroeter, M. L. (2021). *Beyond attention, executive function & memory – resocializing cerebral small vessel disease.* Alzheimers Dement. doi: 10.1002/ alz.12391

Schroeter, M., Kynast, J., Villringer, A. and Baron-Cohen, S. (2021). *Face Masks Protect From Infection but May Impair Social Cognition in Older Adults and People With Dementia.* Frontiers in Psychology, 12.

Thyrian, J. R., Kracht, F., Nikelski, A., Boekholt, M., Schumacher-Schönert, F., Rädke, A., et al. (2020). *The situation of elderly with cognitive impairment living at home during lockdown in the Corona-pandemic in Germany.* BMC Geriatr. 20:540. doi: 10.1186/s12877-020-01957-2

Zheng, G., Wang, Y., Wang, X. (2008). *Chronic hypoxia-hypercapnia influences cognitive function: A possible new model of cognitive dysfunction in chronic obstructive pulmonary disease.* Medical Hypotheses, 71(1), pp.111-113.

Chapter 11

Masks and cases

Images:

Horowitz, D. (2020). Horowitz: *CDC study: 85% of COVID-19 cases in July were people who often or always wear masks.* TheBlaze. Available at: https://www.theblaze.com/op-ed/horowitz-cdc-study-covid-masks (Accessed 21 July 2022).

Weiss, Y. (2020). *These 12 Graphs Show Mask Mandates Do Nothing To Stop COVID.* The Federalist. Available at: https://thefederalist.com/2020/10/29/these-12-graphs-show-mask-mandates-do-nothing-to-stop-covid/ (Accessed 21 July 2022).

Chapter 12

Mass formation, hypochondria and hysteria

21st Century Wire (2022). *An Unsettling Realization: 'Mask Zealots are Sadistic People'* - 21st Century Wire. 21st Century Wire. Available at: https://21stcenturywire.com/2022/04/26/an-unsettling-realization-mask-zealots-are-sadistic-people/ (Accessed 29 July 2022).

Abrams, A. (2017). *The Psychology Behind Racism. Psychology Today.* Available at: https://www.psychologytoday.com/intl/blog/nurturing-self-compassion/201709/the-psychology-behind-racism (Accessed 29 July 2022).

Brodkin, K. (2005). *Xenophobia, the State, and Capitalism.* American Ethnologist, vol. 32, no. 4, 2005, pp. 519–520.

Bronner, S. E. (2018) From Modernity to Bigotry. Critical Theory and Authoritarian Populism, edited by Jeremiah Morelock, vol. 9, University of Westminster Press, London, 2018, pp. 85–106.

Desmet, M. (2022). *The psychology of totalitarianism.* White River Junction, VT: Chelsea Green.

Klein, A. (2018). *Fear, more than hate, feeds online bigotry and real-world violence.* The Conversation. Available at: https://theconversation.com/fear-more-than-hate-feeds-online-bigotry-and-real-world-violence-106988 (Accessed 29 July 2022).

Kopala, M. (2022). *When the Whole World Goes Mad: Mattias Desmet's The Psychology of Totalitarianism* | C2C Journal. C2cjournal.ca. Available at: https://c2cjournal.ca/2022/07/when-the-whole-world-goes-mad-mattias-desmets-the-psychology-of-totalitarianism/ (Accessed 29 July 2022).

Lerner, M. (1969) *Respectable Bigotry.* The American Scholar, vol. 38, no. 4, 1969, pp. 606–617

Manzotti, R. (2020). *Il nuovo bigotto (volgarmente detto "restacasista martire"): Io sono meglio di te perché godo di meno* - LeoniBlog. LeoniBlog. Available at: https://www.leoniblog.it/2020/05/06/il-nuovo-bigotto-volgarmente-detto-restacasista-martire-io-sono-meglio-di-te-perche-godo-di-meno/ (Accessed 29 July 2022).

Mascolo, M. (2019). *Why "Stop Bigotry" Won't Stop Bigotry.* Psychology Today. Available at: https://www.psychologytoday.com/gb/blog/values-matter/201909/why-stop-bigotry-won-t-stop-bigotry (Accessed 29 July 2022).

McCord, W. et al. (1960). *Early Familial Experiences and Bigotry.* American Sociological Review, vol. 25, no. 5, 1960, pp. 717–22.

Pies, R. W. (2007). *Is Bigotry a Mental Illness?* Psychiatric Times. Available at: https://www.psychiatrictimes.com/view/bigotry-mental-illness (Accessed 29 July 2022).

Pies, R. W. (2018). *Why bigotry is a public health problem.* Medicalxpress. com. Available at: https://medicalxpress.com/news/2018-11-bigotry-health-problem.html (Accessed 29 July 2022).

Thomas, J. M. (2014). Medicalizing Racism. Contexts, vol. 13, no. 4, 2014, pp. 24–29.

Chapter 13

Masks and death

Fögen, Z. (2022). The Foegen effect. Medicine, 101(7), p.e28924.

Jones, W. (2022). *Mask Study Finds No Impact on Covid Infections From Mask-Wearing and an INCREASE in Deaths.* The Daily Sceptic. Available at: https://dailysceptic.org/2022/04/30/mask-study-finds-no-impact-on-covid-infections-from-mask-wearing-and-an-increase-in-deaths/ (Accessed 31 July 2022).

Kisielinski, K., Giboni, P., Prescher, A., Klosterhalfen, B., Graessel, D., Funken, S., Kempski, O. and Hirsch, O. (2021). *Is a Mask That Covers the Mouth and Nose Free from Undesirable Side Effects in Everyday Use and Free of Potential Hazards?.* International Journal of Environmental Research and Public Health, 18(8), p.4344.

Morefield, S. (2022). *New Study Alleges Mask Mandates Associated With Increased Covid Death Rate.* Townhall. Available at:

https://townhall.com/tipsheet/scottmorefield/2022/06/05/new-study-mask-mandates-associated-with-increased-covid-death-rate-n2608241 (Accessed 31 July 2022).

Spira, B. (2022). *Correlation Between Mask Compliance and COVID-19 Outcomes in Europe.* Cureus.

Winters, N. (2022). *Mask Mandates Caused MORE COVID Deaths, Study Alleges.* The National Pulse. Available at: https://thenationalpulse.com/2022/05/26/counties-with-mask-mandates-had-higher-covid-19-death-rates/ (Accessed 31 July 2022).

Chapter 14

Conclusions

Dodsworth, L. (2021) A State of Fear. London, Pinter&Martin

Kisielinski, K., Giboni, P., Prescher, A., Klosterhalfen, B., Graessel, D., Funken, S., Kempski, O. and Hirsch, O. (2021). *Is a Mask That Covers the Mouth and Nose Free from Undesirable Side Effects in Everyday Use and Free of Potential Hazards?*. International Journal of Environmental Research and Public Health, 18(8), p.4344.

Youtube.com (2022). *They're Keeping Fear in Our Face, Literally! The REAL Reason They Want Us Wearing Masks*. Available at: https://www.youtube.com/watch?v=P9Shm2oB9sc (Accessed 31 July 2022).

Lightning Source UK Ltd.
Milton Keynes UK
UKHW052230191022
410720UK00009B/57

9 781739 156947